Detox *for* Life

Detox *for* Life

How to Minimize Toxins and
Maximize Your Body's Ability to Heal

DR. DAN NUZUM AND GINA NUZUM-OROZCO

Detox *for* Life

ISBN (paperback) 978-1-941420-31-7
ISBN (hardcover) 978-1-941420-32-4
Library of Congress Control Number: 2017952498

Lead Editor: Kevin Mullani
Editors: Jennifer Regner, Mindy Hubbard, Maryanna Young, Stephanie Mullani
Project Management Support: Aloha Publishing
Cover & Interior Design: Tru Publishing
Recipe Photos: Alyssa Carrera (Orelle Photography), Allie Litterer
Illustrations: Victoria Hilles

Published by Tru Publishing

TruPublishing.com

First Printing, 2017
Printed in the United States of America

To our angels in heaven:

Grandma Christine Mitchell and our son Angelo.

Your profound influence lives forever in our hearts.

CONTENTS

FOREWORD..IX

INTRODUCTION..1

PART 1: STABILIZE

CHAPTER 1—WE LIVE IN A TOXIC WORLD 7

CHAPTER 2—TOXINS IN OUR AIR 11

CHAPTER 3—TOXINS IN OUR WATER 19

CHAPTER 4—TOXINS IN OUR FOOD 27

CHAPTER 5—TOXINS IN PERSONAL PRODUCTS..............................41

PART 2: DETOXIFY

CHAPTER 6—HOW TOXINS AFFECT YOUR BODY..............................53

CHAPTER 7—BEFORE YOU DETOX..63

CHAPTER 8—SIDE EFFECTS OF DETOXING.................................73

CHAPTER 9—NUTRITIONAL SUPPLEMENTS 83

CHAPTER 10—DETOX PROTOCOLS...95

PART 3: FORTIFY—Detox Diet Recipes

RECIPE INTRODUCTION...117

   JUICES 119

   SMOOTHIES...135

   BREAKFAST 147

   SNACKS, DIPS & SAUCES 161

   SOUPS 177

   SALADS 195

   ENTRÉES 211

   PATIENT SUBMITTED RECIPES 233

ADDITIONAL RESOURCES.. 243

Over the course of 368 days, I lost my father, grandfather and uncle from cancer. My father died because of the surgery he underwent to remove the cancer, not the disease itself. This caused me to question, why, after more than 100 years, are we still using treatments for diseases such as this that are as dangerous as the ailment itself. Over the next several years, I lost another grandfather, one grandmother, a cousin and my mother … all due to cancer or its barbaric "treatments." Disease has devastated my family and as a result, my wife, Charlene, and I are rearing children that will never know their grandmother or grandfather.

As tragic as this story is, if these events had never occurred, I would never have left my job as a CPA and begun a lifelong dedication to finding natural ways to treat cancer. I would not have authored best-selling books, or co-founded the now internationally known documentary series *The Truth About Cancer*. I have researched natural medicine for over two decades now and will always support those who reveal the truths about disease and healing as a whole. Believe me, these truths need to be revealed.

According to cancer.org, approximately 600,000 people will die from cancer this year in the United States. According to the Centers for Disease Control, another 630,000 people will die from heart disease, 155,000 from respiratory disease, 110,000 from Alzheimer's disease and 80,000 from diabetes. It's clear that disease is a serious epidemic in our country. It is also clear that the current "solutions" we are utilizing to combat these diseases are not working at an acceptable level.

Albert Einstein once said, "No problem can be solved from the same level of consciousness that created it." Our country has created a massive reliance on allopathic modalities and pharmaceutical drugs that are only perpetuating more problems. Our culture needs to wake up from this current trend that creates a "pill for every ill" and remember that our bodies were created with the ability to heal. Because of my family's experience with disease, I can say without hesitation that I have been able to surround myself with some of the smartest, most effective healers and educators around the world, and I am grateful to call many of them my friends.

Dr. Daniel Nuzum is one of those healers and educators that I met for the first time when I interviewed him for The Quest for the Cures. His track record of healing patients naturally from all types of disease initially attracted me to interview him, but once I learned more about Doc Nuzum, I realized what a rare resource he is in more ways than just practicing naturopathic medicine. He is a former toxicologist, professor, scientist and researcher. He holds seven PhDs in various medical fields and three additional doctorates. He is one of the top formulators for natural supplements in the world and plays a major role in formulating and consulting for many supplement companies. Bottom line, when "Doc" (as I affectionately call him) asked me to write a foreword for his new book that helps educate people on how to naturally heal themselves and take care of their bodies, I jumped at the chance.

I've known Doc and his wife Gina now for many years and couldn't imagine a more qualified husband and wife team to help people understand the importance of detoxification in the healing process. Doc Nuzum's track record as a Naturopath, educator and formulator uniquely qualifies him to teach the general population how they can best support their bodies to be efficient at healing disease. I am also a big believer that if you want to be healthy, you must eat healthy. So, it is perfect that Gina is providing healthy recipes to help guide readers as to how they can shift their dietary habits as well. The combination of the education and detox protocols from Doc Nuzum, and the recipes for healthy eating by Gina make *Detox for Life* a critical resource for everyone interested in optimizing their health.

What motivates me even more regarding this book is that if readers follow the healing process presented by Doc Nuzum—stabilize, detoxify and fortify—their families may be able to avoid some of the pain and suffering that my family had to endure because we didn't have this amazing information. I give it my full endorsement and I am excited to help reach as much of the population as possible with this incredible educational guide.

Read this book in its entirety and share it with friends. You'll be glad you did.

—Ty Bollinger

New York Times Bestselling Author
Co-Founder of www.TheTruthAboutCancer.com

ACKNOWLEDGMENTS

Gina and I are grateful for the love and support of our children, friends, and families.

Gina would like to thank her mother for spending time with her in the kitchen, teaching her how to use whole foods in the creation of healing recipes. She wishes to thank her father for teaching her to look for true riches inside people's hearts. From both parents, she learned how to have faith in God and give from the heart–in all circumstances.

I'm grateful for experiencing the love and generosity of family through my parents adopting and raising 32 children—most with special needs—in addition to me. My siblings were like my first patients, as I was able to participate in and witness their profound growth and healing.

Despite our chaotic household, my mother accomplished her PhD and successfully healed MS in her body by studying and applying natural medicine. Her patience and perseverance were a powerful combination for a child to witness. The support of my father throughout all of our challenges and triumphs, as well as his wisdom, stay with me to this day. Together, both my parents achieved multiple degrees of black belts and continue to be a source of inspiration.

We appreciate the opportunity to cry, laugh, learn, and grow with our patients as they bravely face and overcome their health challenges. They inspire us to keep bringing this healing work to our future patients and to the world.

We give thanks to God for the ability to do this work, and for His guidance and protection on our path.

Sincere gratitude to Ty Bollinger and his wife Charlene for their dedication to spreading important health information so that humanity may experience a revolution in healing.

Finally, we wish to thank Tru Publishing for producing and publishing this book, as well as all those who helped make *Detox for Life* a reality.

You have cancer.

These are words that nobody wants to hear. If you have heard these words, you understand what an impact an affliction like this can have on your life and those around you. The word cancer can be replaced with the name of any serious disease, but the emotional and physical impact will be the same—it's devastating.

One concept, critical to understand, is that people don't suddenly get cancer—or any disease—they develop them over time. *Something* happened that crippled the body's natural ability to defeat illness. This "something" is a combination of nutritional deficiency and toxin overload that in time overwhelmed the body. Typically, your body can identify toxins and adapt by eliminating them through various detox channels such as the liver, skin, kidneys, blood and lymphatic system. When the toxic load becomes too much for the body to eliminate, it begins to accommodate the toxins by storing them. Accommodation of the toxins is what sets the stage for disease. The good news is, everyone has the ability to heal—even when they are overwhelmed. That said, the capacity to heal depends on each individual and the actions they are willing to take to help their bodies return to its optimal state.

Understand that the process for the body to heal disease is no different than to heal any wound. When you cut yourself on a rusty nail, the first thing you need to do is stop the bleeding—or stabilize the wound. Next, you have to clean dirt and rust out of the wound—or detoxify it. A dirty wound will never heal. It can't. Finally, you can fortify the healing process by covering the wound, keeping it clean, and applying some antiseptic salve. Compare this to the process of healing disease in your body. First, for your body to heal you must stabilize the environment by reducing toxic intake and increasing nutrition. Next, you must clean the buildup of toxins that have accumulated over time through detoxification. Remember, no dirty wound, or body can heal.

Finally, you can fortify your body by eating a nutrient rich diet and taking supplements that help your body's detoxification pathways to work optimally.

Once you understand what is required for the healing process that already exists inside your body to work, you can empower yourself with the knowledge of how to stabilize, detoxify and fortify your body to optimize its ability to heal. That is the purpose of this book.

WHY THIS BOOK?

Detox for Life is designed to be a tool to help you revitalize your own healing process. Every concept presented is based on the tenets of natural medicine. Conventional medicine typically only treats symptoms; it rarely eliminates the source of the problem. My goal as a natural practitioner is to help you heal using the *stabilize, detoxify,* and *fortify* process. So to keep it simple, the book is organized into three parts.

Part one, *Stabilize–Sources of Toxins,* will teach you how to stabilize your body and immediate environment by minimizing your exposure to toxins. Most people realize it is impossible to live a normal life and completely eliminate all exposure to toxins, so this section will help educate you about the most common and dangerous sources that we breathe, ingest, and absorb. It is not meant to frighten you, rather empower you with knowledge. When you understand that daily choices are either building your health or tearing it apart, you can make informed decisions to minimize your toxic exposure.

Part two, *Detoxify–Detox Concepts and Protocols*, will teach you how to apply detox-ification once you have stabilized your body. The most pivotal component in the body's three-step healing process is detoxification. As I've said before, a dirty wound cannot heal. This section will help you further understand why you need to detox, what a detox really is, and how to succeed during and after a detox. Of course, I also provide three detox protocols of various intensity that anyone, regardless of whether this is a new concept or you've been detoxing for years, can benefit from. Even though we consider supplementation to be a critical part of both detoxifying and fortifying, it will primarily be discussed in part two.

The last part of the book, *Fortify–Detox Diet Recipes*, will help you fortify your body with good nutrition. My wife Gina tells me all the time that I am the brains and she is the cook, and thank God for that! I am honored to help educate people, but nobody would want to eat my cooking. This is by no means a complete source for clean recipes, but rather an introduction to get you started preparing healthy, nutritious food.

The key to preserving or improving your health is to minimize toxic exposure and maximize your ability to adapt and heal. My mission is to help you preserve and regain health, as much as you are able, by following the process of healing as I have come to understand it. I have utilized this three-step process with patients for over two decades, and Gina and I have seen thousands of people come back to health. Some of their stories are shared throughout this book to inspire you on your healing journey.

Your body has amazing capabilities to adapt to a pretty harsh world. I invite you to learn more about how to *stabilize, detoxify,* and *fortify* your body, so you can maximize your body's ability to heal.

Thank you for reading!

—Dr. Dan and Gina Nuzum

The most pivotal component in the body's three-step healing process is detoxification.

PART 1: STABILIZE

Sources of Toxins

CHAPTER 1

We Live in a Toxic World

Imagine getting ready to leave on a 20-mile hike and everything you'll need has to fit in a backpack. Knowing you have to carry it on your back, you're torn between bringing the luxuries you're accustomed to, or just the practical things you really need. After very little consideration, you ignore your instincts and start throwing whatever you want into your backpack and wherever it lands, it stays. Of course you pack some food and water, but then you add your laptop, in case you need to get some work done. Then your cell phone, with a solar-powered battery charger. Oh yes, you can't forget to pack a reading light and couple good books in case you're trapped inside your tent on a rainy day. You did it! You jammed everything in your pack. You're feeling pretty good about your choices until you reach the trailhead and throw it on. The pack is very heavy, lumpy, and extremely uncomfortable. The solar powered cell phone charger is jutting into your spine, and you start to wonder about your choices. It is going to be a long, hard hike.

Now—imagine that the excess things in your backpack are toxins. Toxins from choices you make simply living your life and doing the things you do, day in and day out. You don't think adding a little fast food here and some cell phone EMFs there will be a big deal. But it all adds up.

TOXINS ARE ALL AROUND US

Toxins are present in our food, air, water, soil, skin care, and just about everything we use, or encounter in daily life. According to the National Toxicology Program (NTP), there are over 80,000 chemicals registered for use in the United States alone. This number increases annually by roughly 2,000 new chemicals in everyday items such as foods, personal care products, prescription drugs, household cleaners, and lawn care products—a heavy load we were never meant to carry. We have mercury amalgams in our teeth, toxic vaccines, fluoride and chlorine added to our water, radiation from rain, and fallout from Fukushima. In addition, these multiple toxins combine with each other to form compounds that are even more toxic.

The human body possesses the ability to defend itself against these unhealthy foreign substances, but only to a degree. We are bombarded by more toxic materials than we can reasonably metabolize and eliminate. When compromised over and over again by daily infiltrations that are impossible to completely escape, the body cannot eliminate the toxins as fast as they are coming in, and it becomes overtaxed. The defense system of the body is smart enough to know that toxins are bad, so it tries to store them in the "safest" possible places, like fat cells, the lymph system, and other areas that won't affect critical functions of the body. In some cases, it surrounds the toxins with fluid to dilute them, making them less toxic, but this creates chronic inflammation. Eventually, as more and more toxins accumulate in our bodies and the "safe" storage areas overflow, they create chaos and interrupt all kinds of normal functions in the body. One of these functions is nutrient absorption.

NUTRIENT DEFICIENCY LEAVES YOU VULNERABLE TO MORE TOXINS

Accommodating toxins by storing them begins a vicious cycle when it comes to nutrient absorption. Many of our cells uptake nutrition via receptor sites within the cell. These sites are designed to receive very specific nutrients that different types of cells require to function. Some toxic elements just happen to be a perfect fit in many of the same receptor sites that absorb nutrients. A perfect example is when your body is exposed to heavy metals: mercury fits in zinc receptor sites, aluminum fits into magnesium receptor sites, arsenic into selenium receptor sites, and lead into calcium receptor sites. These toxic elements block good minerals from being absorbed by the body and create deficiencies.

When your body is nutrient deficient, it becomes more vulnerable to disease and increasingly susceptible to absorb more toxins. In a sense, you become a toxin sponge.

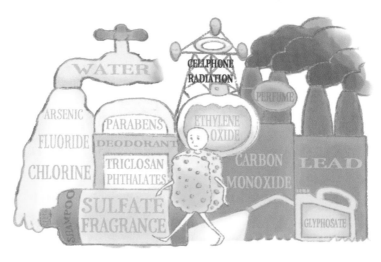

Your body no longer functions in sync and struggles to keep up. When your body is so burdened by trying to eliminate toxins and deal with their side effects, your immune response is greatly hindered.

YOUR BODY CAN'T KEEP UP AND BECOMES OVERDRAWN

The three primary filtration systems that rid your cells of foreign and toxic substances are the liver, kidneys, and lymphatic system. These filters are connected to so many different functions in your body that when one system is compromised, not only is that organ affected, but the body's entire system can be affected. Diseases are caused by the disruptive effect that accumulated toxins have on the body's natural defense mechanisms. Not only are these systems overburdened by the onslaught of toxins, they also take on all the accumulated waste of the toxins themselves. This waste material creates an environment perfect for fungal overgrowth and parasitic infections, wreaking further havoc in your body's systems. In this overloaded state, these defense mechanisms simply can't keep up and the entire immune response is affected.

When the entire immune response has been compromised, sickness and disease find a way in: thyroid crisis, leaky gut, different types of cancers, fatty liver, polycystic kidney, and lymphedema to name a few. You don't have to have a serious disease to realize your immune system is compromised. It may be something much simpler such as frequent colds and flus, headaches, allergies, low energy, lack of mental clarity, or even acne. In many cases, by the time a real disease is present, like diabetes or cancer, you can look back and see that your body has been signaling you for years. Just as a cancerous tumor can take five to seven years to form, toxic build-up happens slowly over time until your body is overwhelmed.

At all times, you are either building your health, or you are tearing it down.

Think of your overall health as a bank account—let's call it your health account. When you take good care of your body by eating whole, organic foods, or by drinking clean water, you are making deposits into your health account. Your body needs these positive deposits to stay operational, just like your household needs a positive balance in your bank account. When you drink too much, spray glyphosate on your weeds, or eat fast food, you are making withdrawals from your health account. At all times, you are either building your health, or you are tearing it down. As I've already stated, it's impossible to eliminate all toxic exposure, but it's critical that you maintain a positive balance so you don't overdraft your account. When your health account becomes overdrawn—huge fees kick in. The toxic debt that is created can quickly get out of hand and the accumulation can become unbearable. Much like the time it takes you to pay back interest and fees for financial debt, it takes your body time to clean itself and to heal.

Remember, the first step in the healing process is to stabilize. Just as we must stop bleeding to stabilize a wound, we must minimize toxic exposure and increase healthy deposits to stabilize our health account.

EDUCATE YOURSELF TO STABILIZE

At some point in your life, you have probably heard that you need to put pressure on a wound to stop the bleeding, right? You most likely learned this from your parents the first time you fell off a bike, or something similar. You were educated with this basic first aid information and probably applied it more than once since.

My goal in the next few chapters is to educate you on what to put in your pack and what to leave out for that long hike we call life—in other words, how to stabilize your body and immediate environment.

These chapters will reveal the sources of the most common toxins in the air, water, food, and commonly used products. If you understand where toxins come from, you will have the knowledge required to make decisions that will reduce your toxin intake and support your health, ultimately optimizing your ability to heal. Of course, solutions on how to minimize your exposure to toxins will be provided along the way as well. So take a deep breath, and dive right in to the next chapter to learn all about the toxins in our air.

CHAPTER 2

Toxins in Our Air

Have you ever planned an outdoor excursion, small or large, only to find out on your way there that all roads north are closed due to poor air quality? Before we can even think about what to pack for our hike, we must think about elements that are a little harder to control.

The average person can survive around three weeks without food, depending on various factors. Good to know, especially if you didn't bring enough food for your 20-mile hike. The same person can only survive about seven days without water. But take away air, and the average person will only survive three to five minutes. Oxygen is life—and breathing clean, quality air can directly affect our health.

OXYGEN NEUTRALIZES TOXINS

Our bodies use oxygen to burn sugars and fatty acids in our cells to produce energy. Additionally, oxygen is a key component that the body uses to neutralize toxins and to remove them from the body. These two functions are pretty critical to our health, so it only makes sense that we would want to ensure every breath we take has a high oxygen content. The problem is, as our atmosphere becomes more polluted, the oxygen is literally being choked out of the air. With city pollution, industrial exhaust, and pesticides and herbicides being constantly sprayed outside, some people may never want to leave their home. But is the air inside any better? Actually, it's not.

The air quality indoors is typically worse than outdoors because the toxins stay contained in a smaller area and don't have as much space to disperse. That said, you have a much better chance of stabilizing the quality of the air inside your home than you do outside.

There are simple things you can do right now to improve air quality indoors:

- open your windows to replace stagnant air

- grow indoor plants to help clean the air
- use salt lamps to clear and refresh the air
- use an aromatherapy essential oil diffuser to help clean the air

Additionally, when you are aware of toxins that exist in your home, and what some of the sources for them are, you can drastically reduce the toxic output that you and your family produce, which will ease the burden on your body.

Below is a list of many common air pollutants:

Pathogens

Most simply put, a pathogen is any microorganism that can cause disease. Pathogens include bacteria, viruses, airborne cysts and spores, and parasites. Cysts and spores of many types of parasites can travel long distances in a dormant state until they find a home in your lungs. Parasites sneak their way into the body when your systems have been weakened from toxin overload, attaching themselves to decaying tissue. Living in a big city or on a farm with lots of animals increases your exposure to parasites.

Chemicals

Chemical toxins we breathe are airborne contaminants such as sprayed pesticides, air pollution from car exhaust, and pollution from industrial processes.

Agricultural and Horticultural Sprays

Farms used to be the place to go to get fresh air, but if a farm is nearby, you may be affected by many different toxic sprays being used on that land. Pesticides and herbicides are toxic to humans and should be avoided whenever possible. Look for organic or natural alternatives for use in and around your home.

Product Off-Gassing

Indoor air pollution includes off-gassing chemicals from many different sources. Building materials used to construct your house, like particle board, may off-gas formaldehyde. Mattresses, especially memory foam mattresses, contain formaldehyde, benzene, and naphthalene.

Watch out for scented candles and other various products that may contain phenol or paraffin. A common substance used to give candles and cleaning products a lemony scent is called limonene. On its own, limonene is not considered harmful, but when mixed with other airborne elements it can form formaldehyde.

Cleaning Products

Cleaning products typically contain numerous toxins. Pay attention to the ingredients in what you're using on a day-to-day basis. Laundry detergents, especially scented detergents, and dryer sheets contain formaldehyde and up to 25 volatile organic compounds (VOCs: organic compounds that are resistant to chemical, photolytic, and biological decomposition, and accumulate in the environment). Also beware of the following cleaners: toilet bowl cleaners that contain chlorine bleach; oven cleaners that contain corrosive alkalis (also called caustics); furniture polish that contains hydrocarbons (VOCs); and window cleaners that contain ammonia or rubbing alcohol.

Plastics

Plastics are everywhere and the chemicals used to make them tend to act as hormone disruptors. They primarily affect the thyroid and sex hormones. The most important thing to know is that when plastics are scratched or heated, they release toxins. The most notable toxins in plastic are bisphenol A (BPA), diethylhexyl phthalate, and many other phthalates. Plastic products manufactured prior to 1979 may also contain polychloronated biphenyls (PCBs). So if you use a plastic spatula on something hot, or pour soup in a plastic bowl, or drink water from a hot plastic water bottle left in the car—you will be ingesting toxins from chemicals that made that particular item.

It is almost impossible to get rid of all plastic but there are definitely ways to minimize exposure in the home by replacing plastic utensils, dishes, and storage containers with wood or stainless steel. And please use glass or stainless steel bottles for water.

Mold

Mold microorganisms play an essential role in our environment. We need them outdoors, but not indoors. Molds growing in your home create spores that can easily become airborne while trying to clean. Once ingested, mold can cause inflammation in your body, brain fog, memory and senility issues, gut issues, digestive issues, ear, nose and throat issues, changes in eyesight, and ringing in ears.

If you suspect mold in your home, I urge you to get it inspected to know for sure. Most disaster clean-up companies have a mold specialist that can test your home properly. You can also buy small test kits at big box stores, but they are very inaccurate. Your health will be severely compromised if there is a significant amount of mold in your house, so do not take mold lightly.

SIMPLE STEPS YOU CAN TAKE TO REDUCE YOUR EXPOSURE TO AIRBORNE TOXINS

Airborne toxins can be more difficult to avoid than those in water or food, but you can take control of your environment in your home and work space.

Choose Cleaner Air

- Choose to improve ventilation when working with chemicals such as paint, adhesives, or cleaning products. Go outside whenever possible, open windows or doors, and use exhaust fans when in any enclosed area.

- Choose low VOC (volatile organic compound) paints, varnishes, and stains.

- Choose to buy unscented, organic personal care and household cleaning products. Or make your own (see below). Avoid all commercial fragrance products that pollute your indoor air.

- Choose to add sources of negative ions and houseplants to your indoor environment, and use only essential oils for aromatherapy.

- Choose to live away from agricultural or industrial environments whenever possible. Be aware of local government spraying programs for mosquitos or noxious weeds so you can close your windows to minimize exposure. Use organic pest control measures in your own yard.

Choose Nontoxic Cookware and Utensils

- Choose to reduce or eliminate use of nonstick pans for cooking. If you cannot replace your cookware right away, make sure not to overheat it and ventilate the area well when cooking. A safer option for cookware is cast iron.

- Choose to eat foods that haven't been heated in a plastic container. Use wooden or stainless steel utensils, and glass containers to store food.

MAKE YOUR OWN CLEANERS

You can make effective household cleaners using the right kind of clean ingredients. I recommend these effective, natural, nontoxic ingredients:

- Baking soda
- Vinegar
- Lemon juice
- Hydrogen peroxide

A mixture of vinegar, water, and lemon juice is one effective all-purpose cleaner that leaves your house smelling fresh.

Disinfectant Room Spray

- 10 drops eucalyptus essential oil
- 6 drops rosemary essential oil
- 6 drops orange essential oil
- 2 drops peppermint essential oil
- 2 drops tea tree essential oil

Mix the essential oils with 4 ounces of distilled water in a container with a fine mist spray atomizer. Shake well and mist around the room to maintain a healthy atmosphere.

Bathroom Disinfectant Cleaner

- 4 ounces white vinegar
- 8 ounces distilled water
- 10 drops tea tree essential oil
- 10 drops orange essential oil
- 5 drops rosemary essential oil
- 2 teaspoons Castile liquid soap

Combine ingredients in a spray bottle. Use to disinfect areas in bathroom.

Fresh Breath Mouthwash

- 2 drops of peppermint essential oil
- 1 drop of tea tree essential oil
- 1 teaspoon Equalizer Concentrate
- 1 teaspoon raw honey
- 4 ounces distilled water

Mix honey with essential oils in a 4-ounce container with a lid, add a small amount of warm distilled water and mix until honey is dissolved. Add remaining water. Shake well before use. Swish a small amount in your mouth and spit out. Do not swallow.

Buy Organic

Natural food or health food stores will have cleaning supplies and soaps that are free of fragrances and toxic chemicals. They contain natural compounds that do a great job of cleaning your home, clothing, and your body. We provide a list of products that we recommend on DrNuzum.com, under the "Detox Tools" tab.

The above list of sources for toxins and ways to reduce some of your airborne pollutants is by no means complete. Rather, it is intended to highlight some of the worst offenders and help you begin to shape the way you think about your role in breathing clean air. You can choose cleaner air! The hike is already challenging enough because of your overloaded pack. It doesn't have to be harder because of compromised air in your home—the same goes for compromised water.

Patient Story

Bio-toxin Illness Due to Black Mold and Pesticide/Chemical Exposure

Seven years ago, my family and I moved into a house that backed up to a farmer's field and irrigation canal. From the first week that we were in the house, I began to get sick. It started with yeast infections, and then my perfect 28-day menstrual cycle was thrown completely off track. This kicked off nearly six straight years of a nightmare straight out of some kind of science fiction novel.

We later learned this "sick house" was contaminated with toxic black mold due to the irrigation canal water that was contaminated with pesticide runoff and leeching into the foundation and walls of the house. There was also ongoing pesticide spraying on the fields that drifted onto our property and into our open windows. Our whole family was being chemically poisoned but it took us over a year to learn this. In the meantime, we suffered greatly.

Here were some of the effects I experienced: severe fatigue, brain fog, ear infections, flu-like symptoms, sore throat, cold sores, vision problems, itching, sometimes burning eyes, uncontrollable coughing spasms that had me coughing up blood and required steroid inhalers to calm, severe constipation and bleeding hemorrhoids, sharp shooting pains in my legs and arms, muscle spasms, numbness in my limbs, and what felt like electrical shocks shooting through my breasts which became permanently painful, tender and swollen. My gallbladder, although clear of stones, had become petrified and needed to be removed. I didn't know it at the time but black mold eats away at the connective tissue in the body. I had dislocated a rib in the moldy house while doing simple jumping jacks, and had also torn the sphincter of Oddi (a muscle in the area of the pancreas and gallbladder) from lifting semi-heavy items. This likely led to compromising blood supply to the gallbladder.

My husband experienced the most intense migraines ever felt that would leave him up for several hours in the night pacing the floor. He also started experiencing severe restless legs at night.

Our daughter had patches of strange looking skin rashes in several different places on her body–legs, bottom, stomach. She was still in diapers at the time and would cry and writhe in pain from the rash that was predominantly in the areas covered by diapers.

Our son experienced frequent bloody noses and the whites of his eyes eventually turned red and watered a great deal. It looked as though his eyes were starting to almost swell shut, and he eventually began to get white bumps around them which looked like pustules that needed to burst.

During the course of the two years we lived in the house, I had seen a total of 12 different doctors in three different states to try and help my family get a solid diagnosis and heal. The consensus was reached that it was something in our environment we were being exposed to, and that we needed to move out of the house immediately. We did, but the damage had been done and now we had to heal from it and no doctor I met up to that point knew how to help me.

It took several years after we had moved out of the house before I watched an episode of *The Truth About Cancer* and heard Dr. Nuzum being interviewed. He thoroughly explained the process by which the body heals, and which organ systems need to detox, and in what order. I thought, "I need to find this guy!" I got on the TTAC email list and started receiving articles where Dr. Nuzum explained some of these things further. I couldn't believe my luck to discover that he was located and practicing in MY state!

From my first appointment with him, he provided a tremendous sense of calm. He understood fully what was happening in my body, and was the first person who knew how to help my entire family clear the toxic black mold from our systems so that we could begin to heal.

We began with a specific probiotic (S. boulardii) to help clear the mold and several of Dr. Nuzum's supplements. Within days, we started to notice improvements. The first thing I noticed was that my kids were missing less days of school due to illness. Every winter for six years was hard on the whole family since the black mold and inhaled chemical pesticides left our lungs severely compromised. This past year—after about five months on the supplements—we experienced our first winter since being exposed that nobody came down with a respiratory illness! And a totally unexpected side effect of doc Nuzum's supplements was that my eye doctor said my eyes were getting "younger" and I now needed a lower strength prescription—lower than what I had for nearly 2 decades!

I have since done many rounds of Doc Nuzum's healing detox protocols and have found tremendous support in Dan and Gina's Facebook group. Their positivity and encouragement has meant the world to me and has helped me to continually experience positive shifts in my health. I have learned to love preparing incredibly healthy plant-based meals for my family. From where I started to where I am today, I would not have thought it was even possible to reclaim and rebuild my health to the degree that I have.

My family and I still take Dr. Nuzum's supplements as they continue to reverse damage from the chemical poisoning we experienced. The more formulations we have tried that Dr. Nuzum has been involved in creating, the better we feel.

Now my family has the health that we need to not only survive each day, but to actually thrive and enjoy life again.

—Stephanie M.

CHAPTER 3

Toxins in Our Water

An essential tool for being in nature for long periods of time is a water filter—one of those light, flexible bags with a built-in filter, meant for purifying lake or river water. Having a source of clean, pure water is essential to your body's ability to receive nutrition. One of the quickest ways to begin stabilizing your body is by drinking clean, pure water.

In my definition, the human body is made up of the same components as dirt. Dirt is nothing more than water, microbes, and elements of the periodic table that make up the minerals in soil and carbon-based organic matter. These same chemical elements are the basic building blocks of every cell structure in the human body. Restated, our bodies contain water: water hydrates us, and floats food and waste. Our bodies contain microbes: microbes play critical roles in our lives and health. And our bodies contain the periodic table: every one of us has a different configuration of the periodic table. In this trio of components, water is the medium in which everything moves, transporting nutrients to the cells and carrying waste away from the cells.

WATER'S ROLE IN YOUR BODY

Making up approximately 60 percent of your body, water is essential for optimal health. It plays many important roles that become impeded if our source of water is not pure. Water is one of the primary building blocks of every cell. It helps our bodies digest and metabolize food, it becomes fluid that lubricates joints and protects our brain, spinal cord and organs, and it acts as a conductor and travel system for nutrients while eliminating toxins from the body. Needless to say, water is critical to almost every function in our body.

Many health conditions can be drastically improved if people drink enough water. Not only does water activate your filtration system, it also helps the lymphatic system (your body's sewer system) to flow. Without enough water, your cells, tissues, and organs cannot get rid of all of their waste.

Your body also uses water to dilute toxins in your body. The more toxins you have, the more water it takes to dilute them. Think about this in relation to obesity. The body's response to toxicity is swelling. The body will dilute toxic materials into parts per million. The more parts per million you have, the more water it takes to dilute that, and the more girth and size you carry. Not only do you lose girth by getting rid of the swelling through detoxification, you're also stimulating all your metabolic processes.

Also, microbes in your gut drink half of the water that you consume. If you drink 64 ounces of water in a day, your "bugs" (the microbes in your gut) are getting 32 ounces. That's half! And you get the rest. So remember, you are sharing your water.

Because microbes also move around in this water and minerals float in it, it's important this water is clean and pure. When your water is clean and viable, it allows for efficient transportation of nutrients inside each cell. But if your water is contaminated by toxins, transportation is disrupted and nutrients are displaced. For example, if minerals are floating in dirty water, the contaminants will disrupt and displace the minerals: mercury will displace zinc; arsenic will displace selenium; and lead will displace calcium. Moreover, water contaminated with pollutants does not efficiently break down into hydrogen and oxygen when your body requires it, and as a result it does not hydrate effectively. How do you stop this disruption and displacement to further stabilize your body? By drinking the purest water you can drink, which isn't likely to be what's coming out of your kitchen tap.

TOXINS IN OUR DRINKING WATER

Your tap water is likely far from pure if it comes from a municipal source. There are many chemicals found in typical drinking water, far beyond the H2O itself. A three-year study conducted by the Environmental Working Group and reported in 2009 found more than 200 unregulated chemicals in the tap water of 45 states in the US, between 2004 and 2009. These unregulated chemicals included industrial solvents, weed killers, refrigerants, and the rocket fuel component perchlorate.

In toxicology, we find that the toxicity of multiple compounds isn't like simple math where 1+1=2. When each chemical or toxic element is bonded to another chemical or toxic element, the toxicity expands exponentially. The sum is much greater than the parts. This is often the aspect that is overlooked when organizations tell people water is "safe." Each element within the water itself may not be terribly harmful, but the combination of toxic elements is untested and has proven to be very harmful. Many of these elements have been purposefully added to water for various reasons and others find their way into the water supply.

The most commonly added chemicals are listed here:

Aluminum (Al)

Aluminum is not considered toxic as an element and is therefore not considered harmful if ingested, unless it exceeds certain levels (.05–2.0 mg/L depending on state standards). At these levels, it is considered a neurotoxin and linked to adverse neurological effects.

Antimony (Sb)

Antimony is a chemical that can cause nausea and diarrhea. It's a carcinogen that upsets the digestive system. At high levels (greater than .0006 mg/L), it has been linked to diseases like cancer, heart problems, and ulcers.

Arsenic (As)

Arsenic occurs naturally in our food and water. But it is also an industrial and agricultural pollutant, commonly known as poison. Water that is subject to such conditions has an elevated chance of dangerous levels of arsenic.

Barium (Ba)

Barium finds its way into our drinking water usually through drilling and smelting copper. It is considered unsafe at levels above two parts per million (2 mg/L) and can result in difficulty breathing, heart arrhythmia, stomach irritation, and brain swelling (encephalitis) as well as liver, heart, and spleen damage.

Cadmium (Cd)

Cadmium is considered safe at low levels but when exceeded for relatively short periods of time, the following effects occur: nausea, vomiting, diarrhea, muscle cramps, salivation, sensory disturbances, liver injury, convulsions, shock, and renal failure.

Chlorine (Cl)

Chlorine is a very dangerous toxin that can be poisonous, even in small quantities, in both liquid and gas forms. Chlorine has long been used to disinfect our drinking water because it controls bacteria growth like Ecoli and Giardia. Research has shown that long-term exposure to chlorine leads to the production of free radicals within the body. Free radicals are carcinogenic, and cause tremendous damage to our cells.

Chromium (Cr)

Often referred to as the Erin Brockovich chemical, chromium contamination is created by industrial processes. It is known to cause cancer and is currently found in over 200 million household water taps. Legal limits are set at 10 parts per billion (0.010 mg/L) but currently, those limits are only enforced in California.

Copper (Cu)

Copper is allowable in fairly high concentrates in municipal water supplies, yet it can be extremely harmful to babies and young toddlers.

Fluoride (F)

Fluoride is naturally occurring, particularly in groundwater and in many natural foods. It is also added to water in many communities in order to prevent tooth decay. But fluoride is actually a very dangerous element that bonds with other elements to create toxic compounds. It acts as a corrosive and oxidizes everything it touches and causes other compounds to become corrosive.

Lead (Pb)

There is no known safe level of lead. Therefore, it is important if lead is found in water to consider it contaminated. Lead in drinking water usually comes from contact with corrosive elements, like batteries or outdated plumbing materials. If your infrastructure is outdated, it is particularly important to know if your water contains lead. When corrosive fluoridated water flows through outdated lead pipes, it causes greater erosion and increases contamination. This is exactly what led to the water crisis in Flint, Michigan.

Manganese (Mn)

Manganese is naturally occurring in rocks and minerals and our bodies need it. But when levels become excessive, it causes neurological problems and learning disorders in children.

Nickel (Ni)

Nickel is a metal that occurs naturally in soil and volcanic dust. But high levels of exposure increases the likelihood of cancer. These levels are typically only witnessed in areas where smelting is prominent. There is an old toxicology saying that goes like this, "Where nickel goes, bacterial infection follows."

Nitrate/Nitrite (NO2/NO3)

High levels of nitrates (above 10 mg/L), typically found in waste sites like landfills or sewage processing plants, pose an increased risk of cancer.

Selenium (Se)

Selenium is a metal found in natural ore deposits. It is considered to be a nutrient and has made its way into the water system through petroleum and metal refineries. Unsafe levels (above .05 parts per million (.05 mg/L) cause issues with the nervous system, irritability, peripheral vision, and damage to the liver and kidneys, as well as issues with hair and fingernails.

Uranium(U)

Uranium can break down into a soluble form that can contaminate our drinking water. Drinking water containing uranium can cause kidney problems.

There are other chemicals that we find in water like potassium (K), both as sulfites and salts, but these chemicals have minimal impacts. There are also residues from pharmaceuticals, industrial chemicals, and sewage. Did you realize there's an acceptable amount of sewage that can come out of your faucet?

TOXINS INHIBIT HYDRATION

Water should break off into two gases, hydrogen and oxygen. But if your water is contaminated, it doesn't break off. It stays in a liquid form throughout your whole gut. We've had patients who are drinking tap water and working hard to stay hydrated. Some of them have found themselves in the hospital, only to find out they are dehydrated. How can that be? They've been drinking a gallon or a gallon and a half every day.

The water they are drinking is not actually hydrating their body because it's not the kind of water the body can utilize well. Pure water is the key for nourishment. If you spend efforts and money on taking supplements specific to your needs but you're not drinking good water, your body won't be able to carry the nutrition into your cells. Without good water and nutrition, your cells cannot operate well. And when they don't operate well, they cannot detox. Drinking enough good water will help stabilize your body and amplify the effects of your detox.

Drinking enough water can be a challenge. To start, we recommend you develop a relationship with a glass water bottle. If you use plastic water bottles, get rid of them. They contain chemicals that disrupt your hormones. Be aware that the "BPA Free" label on plastic bottles (BPA stands for bisphenol A) simply means that BPA has been replaced with another chemical, and its safety is unknown.

Drinking enough water every day improves many conditions, so try to follow these daily water intake guidelines based on your body weight:

- 120-160 pounds, drink 64 to 72 ounces
- 160 to 200 pounds, drink 72 to 96 ounces
- 200 pounds or more, drink 100-120 ounces

HOW TO MINIMIZE TOXINS FROM WATER

The most important message is to drink, cook, and bathe in the purest water you can obtain. As I have already highlighted, tap water is highly contaminated. You have no way of knowing what's in your water, but you can take steps to further purify what comes out of your tap with filters or processes designed to remove heavy metals and carbon-based chemicals, including weed killers, solvents, and pharmaceuticals. It's time to add a water filter to that backpack before you find yourself depleted and dehydrated.

We recommend these types of water filtration or purification for drinking and cooking:

Best: Reverse osmosis (RO) filtering. Systems for home use are available, even small units for use at a single sink. RO systems will pull 99 percent of waste out of the water, without adding to your electric bill. They can be obtained at any big box home improvement store or online. Installation is easy and maintenance is minimal. Whole home units are also available, so that all the water in your home is purified. These usually require professional installation, but the expense is worth it for your health. APEC (www.freedrinkingwater.com) is one company that makes great RO systems to fit any budget.

The primary concern with RO water is that it removes minerals too. It is much more important to have pure water in your system than to rely on it to provide your minerals, so we still recommend this method. Also, there are products you can buy to add trace minerals back to your water. Adding a few sprays of Equalizer Concentrate in your glass, or taking Super Earth Energy are both great options to add supplemental minerals. Both products are available at DrNuzum.com.

Next best: Berkey filtration systems (berkeyfilters.com). The Berkey website states a person can utilize almost any outside natural water source and transform it into pure drinking water, all while using a natural method without the use of chemicals or complicated processes. They are less expensive than whole home RO systems, but are comparable in price to under-sink systems. These come in a variety of sizes and are portable.

Most affordable: Purchased distilled water. Even though it is in plastic, it's still better than tap water. Or hire a water service that delivers it in five-gallon jugs. You may have to specifically ask a water supplier for BPA-free bottles as they may not offer them without asking.

The purest water is distilled water. However, water distillation units are not practical or affordable for most people. Plus, the same controversy exists around distilled water because distillation removes all the minerals, similar to reverse osmosis.

Start by purifying the water you drink and cook with, but understand that water you bathe in is also a source of toxin exposure. It is common to find on the internet that our skin is an impenetrable layer designed to keep harmful things out—this is partially true. The fact is that the skin does absorb, or allow in, some elements. Have you seen a commercial for nicotine patches? This obviously wouldn't be a viable solution to stop smoking if we couldn't absorb the chemicals in the patches through our skin.

You can reduce the toxins from your shower or bath by using fairly simple solutions, just as we mentioned for drinking and cooking.

A whole home reverse osmosis system is the most complete option to ensure all showers and tubs are safe from toxins. That said, they are quite expensive and may not be a possibility for everyone. A cheap and simple solution for your shower is to install a filter at the shower head. These may not be as effective as RO systems, but the point is to reduce toxicity as much as possible.

The most important message is to drink, cook, and bathe in the purest water you can obtain.

If you are not a shower person, you can neutralize toxins in your bath with the recipe below:

  1 cup Epsom salts

  1/2 cup baking soda

  5 drops of frankincense essential oil

Combine ingredients, add to water, and let sit for 10 minutes before getting in the tub.

Like breathing clean air, drinking clean water is absolutely critical to stabilizing your immediate environment and your body so you can move efficiently toward better health. In many ways, you can actually control the quality of your water easier than you can control the air you breathe. Through the use of filters and clean containers, as well as the recipe provided to neutralize toxins in the tub, you can take action today to lessen your toxic intake and relieve some of the burden your body carries—even with your next glass of water.

Next, learn how to choose the cleanest, most beneficial foods to put in your pack. Some foods will only weigh you down, but minimizing the toxins in the fuel you eat will lighten your step and give you the energy you need to keep hiking.

Patient Story

Chronic Migraines

When I first met Dr. Nuzum, I had been dealing with chronic migraines (two or three a week) for over 20 years. I was tired, drained, had no energy and thought that I was destined to live with migraines for the rest of my life. I homeschool my two young children as well as participate in many activities outside the home, and dealing with constant migraines put a tremendous strain on trying to live an enjoyable, productive life.

Dr. Nuzum recommended his 2-Week Detox program; I had never done any kind of a detox program before so I wasn't sure what to expect. I did not need to worry. Dr. Nuzum gave me all of the necessary supplements as well as a detailed menu plan and shopping list to help me stick with the detox program. I also had access to a Facebook Group that Doc's wife, Gina, maintains called Detox Your Way to Health. All of these tremendous resources were instrumental to my success while on the program.

The first week was difficult as I adjusted to a new way of eating and drinking, but I had reached a point in my health journey that I was so desperate for relief, I would try anything. The menu plan was so helpful in the detox program. It took away the guess work of what I was supposed to buy and eat and instead gave me hope that I really could get through the two weeks. By the second week, I was feeling FANTASTIC! I was sleeping better, I had energy when I got out of bed in the morning, I had energy throughout the day and… the chronic migraines were GONE. I went from two to three migraines each week to only one migraine during the entire 2-Week Detox and on top of all of that–I lost weight too! It's amazing how the body can repair and heal itself given the proper food and nutritional supplements.

This program has helped our entire family; our energy levels have improved and our weight is at a healthy, maintained level. We sleep better at night and have the desire to be out with friends and exploring in nature rather than just sitting on the couch watching television.

Dr. Nuzum and Gina have helped to transform me into a different person, and for that, I am eternally grateful. My advice to anyone looking at this detox program would be this: Don't wait until you're at the end of your rope like I did. Start your journey to health NOW. And if you feel like you've hit rock bottom, I can tell you from personal experience, there is hope, and these products will change your life. Start your journey of freedom TODAY with Dr. Nuzum's 2-Week Detox; You'll be glad you did.—Tammi D.

CHAPTER 4

Toxins in Our Food

The kitchen is the heart of a home, where everyone naturally gathers. But what would happen if you constantly stuffed waste in the kitchen trash, without ever taking it out? It would overflow. If you continued stuffing your trash, it would spill out where you cook and your kitchen would eventually become toxic. Once your kitchen is toxic, it doesn't operate as well. And if your kitchen doesn't operate well, the rest of your home won't either.

The same concept applies to your body. If you're eating toxic foods, it's like throwing trash into your body. When your body overflows with toxins, its ability to deal with the overflow hinders the operation of other functions—and it can't adapt quickly enough to eliminate them. Food plays a huge role in the stabilization of your body and environment, so this chapter will show you the sources of toxins in your food and why you need to . . . take out the trash.

WE ARE EATING OUR WAY TO ILLNESS AND TOXICITY

Commercially produced foods are full of pesticides, herbicides, waxes, and other noxious chemicals and toxins that our bodies retain within our fat cells, our blood, and our organs. A database maintained by the Food and Drug Administration (FDA) titled, *Everything Added to Food in the United States* (EAFUS) shows a list of nearly 4,000 food additives that are tracked and regulated. Of course, not all of them have been fully tested for toxicity, and it's a safe bet that combinations of the additives have not been tested to see how they react to each other. So if you're consuming food that is already loaded with toxins, you are contributing additional toxic waste that your body must process in order to maintain optimal health.

Your body's favorite place to store toxins is in fat cells. This is evident by looking at a sample of our population at the mall. Count how many thin people you see and you will realize it's a lot easier than counting the ones who aren't thin. In this country, the lack of thin people illustrates two important points:

1. People are swollen and distended, and;
2. This swelling is a result of intoxication.

Fat cells are the normal place for our body to store the toxic waste that hasn't yet been metabolized and eliminated. But in very thin people, toxins are actually stored in the nervous system and organ tissue. Toxins stored in the cells of organs, tissues, and muscles are much harder to detoxify than fat cells. Obviously, this causes even greater problems.

The body has the ability to detoxify itself but it needs nutrient rich, whole foods to do this—the raw materials, the nuts and bolts. If your body has become overwhelmed with toxins from unwholesome food and the environment, it will store that toxic load in fat cells. The body begins to take on extra water and swell in effort to neutralize and eliminate toxic materials. If toxic waste is not eliminated, it accumulates and is diluted with extra water. But the body doesn't always expand outward when it swells. Swelling can occur inwardly before it starts to expand and swell outwardly, so being thin doesn't always point to good health.

The body needs whole foods to sustain health and detoxify.

Your body needs raw materials—nutrients, antioxidants, fiber, prebiotics to feed your gut microbes, and minerals to keep your metabolic processes operating normally. These raw materials are what keep the body's machinery operating smoothly.

The standard American diet (SAD) does not supply the raw materials that organic, whole foods deliver. You must understand that to detoxify your body, improve your health, and maintain your health, you cannot continue to eat the SAD on a daily basis. It cannot sustain you.

HOW TOXIC IS THE STANDARD AMERICAN DIET?

Food in the supermarket may begin in the ground, but by the time it reaches packaging and store shelves, it has been so processed that it has turned into a product, more than a viable food item. It's not a live substance anymore. Eighty to ninety percent of the food you find in grocery stores is processed, packaged, and contaminated with additives, excess salts and sugars, and residues from pesticides and herbicides.

The marketing practices of large companies in the food processing industry have targeted children in a way that has incorporated these processed foods into the daily lives and diets of families in the US. This shift in the average diet of American families has had a long-term destructive effect on our health. Much of these practices began in the mid-1980s when large food companies were purchased by tobacco companies, in an attempt to diversify business models due to the staleness of the tobacco industry. As a result, childhood obesity has tripled since 1980. At $215 billion a year, the cost of obesity (in public and private medical spending and lost productivity) to the US economy is now greater than the cost of smoking. Food companies continue to target their marketing of high-fat (unhealthy fats), high-sugar, and high-sodium (MSG) foods to America's children. They use deceptive and misleading tactics that the tobacco companies used to pursue profit at the expense of US public health.

In 2009, after Congress proposed self-regulation by the food industry of their unethical marketing to children, food companies began an aggressive lobbying campaign through a friendly-sounding organization they created, called the Sensible Food Policy Coalition. The Coalition members included PepsiCo, General Mills, and Kellogg's, along with some large media companies. They work through a law and lobbying firm that also represents a major tobacco company. This was just one among many lobbying front groups that continued to promote the unhealthy sugar and fat laden products that were designed to appeal to children. The results of their efforts are continued profits and, sadly, rising rates of obesity and disease.

A look at how the USDA defines *organically* produced food may help you understand what might be in *non-organic* food:

- Prohibited use of synthetic pesticides and herbicides, petroleum-based fertilizers, and sewage sludge-based fertilizers
- Requirement that animals be given organic feed and have outdoor access
- Prohibited use of artificial coloring, flavoring, and preservatives
- Prohibited use of growth hormones, antibiotics, or animal byproducts fed to livestock animals
- By definition, organic foods must be non-GMO

If you think of the organic food labeling requirements as an indicator of how contaminated conventional food production has become, you will realize that no one benefits from eating food that is produced using non-organic practices. One indicator of the sad state of the American diet, and our resulting health, is the increasing number of food allergies and sensitivities many people are experiencing.

FOOD SENSITIVITIES AND ALLERGIES

If you have a sensitivity or an allergic reaction to a food, that food becomes a toxin for you, causing stress and inflammation. Below are some of the most common sensitivities and allergies our population is dealing with:

GLUTEN

Many people are apparently becoming sensitive to gluten, which has created a long-running, gluten-free diet craze. I often pose the question at medical seminars, "Do people have a gluten allergy or do they have glyphosate poisoning?"

Do people have a gluten allergy or do they have glyphosate poisoning?

Gluten is the protein component of the wheat plant. It has been in our diet for thousands of years. Why is gluten suddenly causing that much damage, or autoimmune conditions, such as celiac disease?

It may be that your body is reacting to the glyphosate (a synthetic compound, herbicide) in gluten, rather than the gluten itself. Gluten is the component in wheat that absorbs all of the pesticides and herbicides that are applied to the plant. Residues from these pesticides and herbicides make people sick. This can happen with GMO or non-GMO wheat. Only organic wheat would not have significant amounts of these residues.

Other than pesticide and herbicide poisoning, it is possible to develop an allergy to a food that you eat too much of with too little variety. For example, suppose you eat oatmeal for breakfast every day and you do that for twenty years. After repeated years of consuming the same thing over and over again, you may likely develop an allergy to oatmeal. If you don't vary your diet to an extent, your body eventually creates a response to foods you eat too much of.

Your gut and digestive tract can also be damaged by antibiotics, heavy metal poisoning, and the toxic effects of some vaccines. In many cases, this damage causes severe allergies to specific foods, including gluten. These harmful effects can leave people unable to metabolize grains—specifically gluten—which causes a lack of the necessary enzymes for metabolizing grain proteins.

When someone has an allergic response, their body has developed a reaction against a specific compound such as gluten. If you have developed a gluten sensitivity, you need to avoid gluten for at least 90 days before your immune response starts to calm down. After that, even exposure to clean gluten may still trigger a response for a while. Detoxification can help with this condition because it cleans out the gut. When your gut is clean, it can recolonize with good bacteria (microbes) that will stop the reactions. But this takes some time, and it emphasizes what I said about the water, the periodic table (your mineral makeup), and the microbes. The microbes run your system. It is imperative that you reorganize your microbes through detox to achieve the right balance of beneficial organisms.

It is imperative that you reorganize your microbes through detox to achieve the right balance of beneficial organisms.

FOOD ADDITIVES

Food additives such as dyes, artificial flavors, and preservatives add to the toxin load contained in processed foods. I already mentioned that there are nearly 4,000 food additives currently tracked by the FDA. We obviously couldn't list them all, but below are some of the most prevalent additives and some of their effects:

Preservatives

Preservatives are low-dose antibiotics. They do exactly the same thing to your gut flora that antibiotics would do—they kill them. So if you eat something that contains preservatives, those preservatives are killing off the good microbes like beneficial fungi and bacteria. When you think of the word antibiotic, think anti-life.

Damage done to your gut flora impacts your ability to absorb nutrients. We know that certain microbes in our gut extract specific nutrients and feed them to the gut wall. Calcium-extracting microbes take the calcium out of your food and plug them into receptor sites in your gut wall so your body absorbs the calcium. If you lose too many calcium-extracting microbes, you don't absorb calcium. Other microbes specialize in extracting other nutrients—so if you eat too many preservatives, you destroy gut microbes that help you obtain nutrients from your food, resulting in nutrient deficiency and digestive dysfunction.

Below is a list of harmful preservatives and food products that contain them:

- Aspartame artificial sweetener—found in diet beverages, Jello, sugar-free gum, drink mixes, baking goods, chewable vitamins, and toothpaste
- High-fructose corn syrup—found in most processed foods, bread, candy, flavored yogurts, salad dressings, canned vegetables, and cereals
- Monosodium glutamate (MSG)—found in Chinese food, many snacks, chips, cookies, seasonings, most Campbell Soup products, frozen dinners, and lunch meats
- Trans fat—found in margarines, chips and crackers, baked goods, and fast foods
- Food dyes (Blue #1, Blue #2, Red #3, Red #40, Yellow #6, Yellow Tartrazine)—found in many processed foods including beverages, canned fruit, candy, and pet foods
- Sodium sulfite—found in wine and dried fruit
- Sodium nitrate/sodium nitrite—found in processed, cured meats including bacon and hot dogs
- BHA and BHT (butylated hydroxyanisole, butylated hydroxytoluene)—found in potato chips, cereal, frozen sausages, shortening, candy, and Jello
- Sulfur dioxide—found in beer, soft drinks, dried fruit, juices, wine, and vinegar

- Potassium bromate—found in bread and related baked goods
- Propyl paraben—muffins, tortillas, and dyes
- Aluminum additives (sodium aluminum phosphate or sodium aluminum sulfate)—baked goods

To avoid food additives, buy organic, whole foods and avoid processed foods whenever possible. For even more information, read my blog post about the "10 Toxic Villains You Can (and Should) Avoid" and the "15 Anti-Inflammatory Foods" that should be part of your diet.

SUGAR: BAD IN SO MANY FORMS

Addiction to sugar is a huge problem in the United States. The adult consumption rate of sugar has increased by 30 percent over the last 30 years. It is everywhere and Americans can't seem to get enough of it.

The American Heart Association recommends that adult women should not consume more than six teaspoons of added sugars a day. For men, nine teaspoons a day. Keep in mind this is added sugar, not naturally occurring sugar in fruits and vegetables. The average American will consume about one hundred pounds of added sugar per year; this is about thirty teaspoons a day.

White sugar is the absolute worst type of sugar. Replace white sugar with natural sweeteners such as honey or coconut sugar. Remember, naturally occurring sweeteners are still a form of sugar, so be careful to not go overboard. Most people don't have a problem avoiding a spoonful of sugar nearly as much as they simply aren't aware of the hidden sugar in so many foods.

A single can of cola contains a little over nine teaspoons of sugar. It is found in salad dressings, pickled foods, soups, and even peanut butter. Some yogurts, which most people consider a healthy breakfast, contain more GMO sugar than a doughnut! Many yogurts marketed for children contain GMO sugar and other GMO ingredients, synthetic vitamins, and food coloring. Products marketed light are also misleading, and possibly even worse, because they have other additives to make up for the lost flavor. Reading the labels of packaged foods is the best way to avoid added sugar to your diet.

Sugar has many different names, so here is what to look for when reading labels:

- Fructose
- Lactose
- Sucrose
- Maltose
- Glucose
- Dextrose
- High fructose corn syrup
- Natural Sweetener

Food products with a significant amount of added sugar:

- Soft drinks, including sports drinks and iced tea
- Flavored coffee drinks
- Flavored yogurt
- Barbecue sauce
- Packaged cereals and granolas
- Protein and cereal bars
- Prepared soups
- Canned fruit
- Canned baked beans
- Ketchup
- Cereals
- Granola bars

Eating sugar-rich foods has terrible effects on your body. Sugar consumption has been linked with breast cancer, heart disease, diabetes, and obesity. It can also have less noticeable negative effects such as inflammation and slowed metabolism. It puts you at risk for chronic illness and disease. Sugar also stresses your adrenal glands by causing inflammation that the body requires cortisol to suppress.

Sugar stimulates areas of our brain that triggers a feel-good feeling. Just like a drug addiction, we start to chase that good feeling and crave it. This sensation is dulled with continued use over time, so we have to eat more and more sugar to get the same feeling. When you cut sugar from your diet, you can experience withdrawal symptoms similar to detoxing from smoking or a drug addiction. Headaches, nausea, and fatigue are common and in some cases, people experience a full-on meltdown. Despite these withdrawal symptoms, eliminating processed and GMO sugar is one of the healthiest things you can do, and soon enough you will re-train your body to get the feel-good feeling from real nutrients.

To help make this transition as smooth as possible, increase your intake of green foods and take the following nutritional supplements:

- Chromium polynicotinate helps the liver be more sensitive to insulin, which improves insulin metabolism. You can find it at health food stores or online.
- Banaba leaf helps with blood sugar balance. You can find it at health food stores or online.
- Cinnamon in capsules helps with blood sugar balance.

- Juniper berry helps with blood sugar balance via kidney clearing of excess blood sugar. You can find it at health food stores or online.

- Magnesium oil helps to metabolize sugars in the body. You can find this on DrNuzum.com.

- Green coffee bean extract improves post-meal blood sugar levels and is beneficial to metabolic and cardiovascular systems, as well as the liver. See our Super Chlorogenic product on DrNuzum.com.

- Cordyceps mushrooms and Rhodiola Rosea support the adrenal and thyroid glands to help battle fatigue. You can get these supplements individually (newchapter.com) or combined in my Super Earth Energy (DrNuzum.com).

- Fulvic acid spray Equalizer Concentrate. You can find this on DrNuzum.com.

If you could implement only one thing from this book (even though I hope you pick many), I would want you to eliminate processed sugar from your diet.

Many conditions such as metabolic syndrome with high cholesterol and high blood pressure, autoimmune disease, chronic fatigue, fibromyalgia, chronic pain, anxiety, depression, ADHD, hormonal imbalances, heart disease, irritable bowel syndrome, and candida overgrowth will be impossible to fully overcome if you are consuming processed sugar.

> If you could implement only one thing from this book, I would want you to eliminate processed sugar from your diet.

The longer you are off sugar, the less you will crave it. I developed the 2-Week Detox program you will find in chapter ten to help you detoxify and to get off refined sugars. In this program, you are required to only use natural sugars such as raw organic honey, raw organic maple syrup, or organic coconut sugar, and no more than 1 to 2 tablespoons in one day. Some fruit is allowed but in small amounts. People that have completed this program have changed their taste buds and continue to only use natural sugars as part of their new lifestyle. Many have come back and said, "Doc, I know what real food taste likes now! And I don't crave sugar like I used to!"

PESTICIDES AND HERBICIDES

Toxins also come from the pesticide and herbicide residues found in conventionally grown crops. On average, a non-organic apple from bud to picking will get exposed to pesticides five times in its growth cycle. Those pesticides don't just fall off the peel of the apple. They get incorporated into the apple itself, and you can't detoxify the apple.

One of the most commonly used herbicides today is glyphosate. Glyphosate residues are present in nearly all GMO foods, as well as in some non-GMO foods.

Glyphosate

Glyphosate is routinely used on GMO crops, but non-GMO foods can also have glyphosate residues because they are sprayed for weeds. Currently, the FDA does not require testing for glyphosate residues in food or the labeling of GMO-containing foods. To be certain you are avoiding glyphosate residues, your only choice is to eat foods labeled as 100 percent organic (and hope the farmer next door is not spraying with it).

The safety of glyphosate has been questioned by many, especially since the World Health Organization's IARC (International Agency for Research on Cancer) ruled that glyphosate is a probable human carcinogen. Proposition 65 is a California law that requires the state to publish a list of chemicals known to cause cancer or birth defects or other reproductive harm. This list must be updated at least once a year and has grown to include approximately 800 chemicals since it was first published in 1987. Glyphosate was added to that list in July 2017 and mandates that any product containing glyphosate to be labeled as a carcinogen. Just prior to this, in June 2017, a lawsuit was filed in federal court in Wisconsin against Monsanto (the maker of Roundup) and Scotts Miracle-Gro (distributor of Roundup) by residents of Wisconsin, Illinois, California, New York, New Jersey, and Florida. The suit alleges that the companies falsely claimed that glyphosate "targets an enzyme that is not found in people or pets." The plaintiffs have claimed that the targeted enzyme is also found in beneficial bacteria inhabiting the intestinal tract of people. These gut bacteria are critical to health and could be killed by ingesting foods with glyphosate residues.

To understand the danger of glyphosate, it's important to know something about the amino acid glycine. Glycine is a component of every tissue in your body and is the smallest essential amino acid. It is an important enabler of the correct folding, or bending, of protein chains to make active enzymes. What is interesting about the glyphosate molecule is that it is a modified form of glycine and can be a glycine analogue, literally taking the place of glycine in body processes. For example, if the DNA that is making proteins accidentally grabs a glyphosate molecule instead of glycine, glyphosate can potentially be incorporated into every protein that's synthesized in your body. If this larger glyphosate molecule is incorporated, the correct folding of the amino acid chain cannot happen, and the enzyme's function is changed or destroyed. This means glyphosate can potentially modify DNA function and prevent DNA repair, which is a critical part of the body's defense against cancer—against mutated DNA. So you can see that the issue of glyphosate on crops is nothing to ignore.

While glyphosate may not be incorporated directly into DNA, its substitution for glycine in your body's enzymes will potentially disrupt normal, critical processes everywhere in your body.

The damage from this herbicide in your body can affect all processes because it can affect any protein your body synthesizes. Enzymes, the "factories" that run your metabolism, are proteins. If glyphosate can be substituted for the essential amino acid glycine in protein synthesis, any enzyme with glyphosate substitution will not operate properly. The malfunctions can potentially cause almost any disease.

Glyphosate residues in food are arguably the greater threat to your health than glyphosate in the air, and everyone who eats the standard American diet is regularly exposed to it.

Glyphosate is present in 70 percent of the water in our country and its favorite cohort is fluoride. It will bind to 80-90 percent of the periodic table as a salt form. Minerals in salt form act like heavy metals. Plants typically modify minerals into a carbon-based ionic form that your body can readily use. GMO plants that are sprayed with glyphosate cannot absorb minerals, nor convert these minerals for your body to use. This makes GMO plants nutrient deficient. When we eat nutrient deficient plants, we become nutrient deficient too. Nutrient deficiency is a separate issue from toxin exposure, but they are closely related.

If the plants you eat are nutrient deficient, so are you.

Your best choice for clean food is 100 percent organic, but there are some conventionally grown crops that don't need significant spraying to grow. These crops can still be a part of your healthy diet.

NUTRIENT DEFICIENCY ENABLES TOXICITY

If food is deficient in nutrients, the people eating the food will also be deficient in nutrients, which increases the likelihood of absorbing toxins. Nutrients block our bodies from absorbing toxins. For instance, mercury can plug into the same receptor sites in our cells as zinc, selenium, and sulfur. So if you're deficient in zinc, selenium, and sulfur while you're being exposed to mercury, it can plug into those empty receptor sites. Once the receptor sites are blocked by toxins, it's hard to get the zinc, selenium, and sulfur in there. It's a nasty cycle.

Many studies have compared nutritional content between organic and conventionally grown fruits and vegetables. Conventionally grown produce tends to grow faster and be larger in size, which can lead to a dilution effect of the available nutrients. In addition to the dilution, GMO plants may only pick up 8-13 nutrients from the soil. On a daily basis, you need 73 different nutrients to function optimally, so if your food has only 8-13, it cannot supply your basic needs.

One comparison revealed that it takes approximately nine conventionally grown apples to make up the nutritional value of one organic apple. The higher cost of organic produce can be more easily justified when you know this.

Labeling of Organic versus Non-GMO Foods

There is a significant difference between "USDA certified organic" and other labeling you will find on food. One often-blurred difference is between organic and non-GMO. Most simply, know that foods labeled organic will always be GMO-free, but non-GMO does not mean the product is organic.

GMO stands for genetically modified organism. It is a seed or plant that has been genetically engineered by scientists for a number of reasons: to withstand large amounts of pesticides or herbicides, to grow at an accelerated rate, to produce more in a shorter lifespan, or to provide other benefits for food production. It is important to note that GMOs are not natural and are a product of scientific engineering.

There has been a big push across the globe to label foods that contain GMOs. Many countries in Europe have banned them from their shelves completely. As a result of the demands of the American consumer, the "Non-GMO Project" was born. The "Non-GMO Project" label was created to notify consumers when a product contains less than 0.9 percent of GMO ingredients. This is not to be confused with an organic labeling. The product could have still been sprayed with pesticides, had antibiotics used in its production, or been exposed to other chemicals used in farming operations.

Organic labeling, as determined by the USDA, prohibits the use of any GMOs or use of synthetic pesticides or herbicides in the growing and processing of the product. However, the USDA regulation only ensures 95 percent of the product is non-GMO. This is why it is important to look for clear labeling that states 100 percent organic.

Packaging

Processed food packaging often contributes toxins to the food it contains. Bisphenol A (BPA) use is one of the most well-known issues with food containers and packaging to date. It is clear that BPA is a widespread contaminant that can be found in the urine of most people. BPA is found in can liners for food and beverages of all types. Foods and beverages that are heated in containers or lined cans made with BPA are likely to contain more BPA than those that aren't heated.

Here is our best advice to avoid this toxin and others that may be in plastic containers:

- Glass, ceramic, and stainless steel are the cleanest materials for containing foods and beverages.
- Glass, ceramic, and cast iron are the cleanest materials for cookware. Stainless steel is better than cookware with non-stick coatings, but it may have other metals that leach into food when heated.
- Never heat foods or beverages in a microwave, or any other way, in any kind of plastic container.

- Avoid eating food or drinking beverages that are packaged in cans or plastic bottles.

- Never follow the "cook-in-the-bag" or "boil-in-the-bag" instructions found on some fresh and frozen food products. Remove them from any plastic packaging and cook them in glass, ceramic, or cast-iron cookware.

Note that some manufacturers have responded with "BPA-free" lined cans and it is unknown what has replaced the BPA in these products. It has a shorter history of use in our food and may be no better than BPA.

THE SAD PLAN ISN'T WORKING

The SAD clearly has become nutrient deficient and contaminated, and does not support your health. From baby formula to pesticide-contaminated, nutrient-deficient foods, the SAD plan is truly a disaster. But there is hope. Eating clean, organic food and taking quality supplements can restore what has SADly been taken from you.

Many patients have done very well in our clinic following my supplement protocols. And those who adopted a clean eating program along with supplements, by far, had the best results. Most who heed this advice wouldn't dream of trading their old ways of eating for the mind and body connection they have now discovered. By integrating a cleaner diet with supplements, you give your body the best, most stable environment for change.

> By integrating a cleaner diet with supplements, you give your body the best, most stable environment for change.

We've already discussed that your body is not receiving adequate nutrition on the SAD, which supplies only 17 out of 73 essential nutrients. Even those 17 remaining nutrients are devalued because of chemicals or artificial ingredients. If you randomly took 80 percent of the nuts and bolts out of your car, would it still run? If so, would you attempt to drive that car?

We believe our country needs a food revolution. A small portion of people are waking up to this movement, and while it's growing, too many are still in the dark. It starts by getting informed and continues with our day-to-day habits.

The good news is that the movement has started and is gaining strength. Many are recognizing the real benefits of eating organic foods. Most grocery stores are even starting to pay attention, making it easier to find quality food. Every time you purchase an organic product, your dollars vote—and that vote is a huge voice.

If you are (and I truly hope so) one of those people, like myself, who wants to learn new things, grow, and enjoy healthy foods that won't jeopardize your health and instead give you a vibrant life, I am excited to take you on this journey of delicious and detoxifying foods.

WHAT YOU CAN DO TO AVOID TOXINS IN FOOD

These are some of the most critical steps you can take to avoid toxins in food:

- Avoid processed foods and beverages of all types.
- Buy organic whenever possible.
- Stay updated on the "clean fifteen," a list of produce that has the lowest levels of pesticides and are relatively safe to eat, even as non-organic. The Environmental Working Group (EWG) maintains this list and updates it frequently.
- Avoid the "dirty dozen," which is another list from the EWG that identifies the most heavily sprayed produce. These vegetables are best purchased as organic to avoid exposure to heavy doses of pesticides.

Read labels and visit the Environmental Working Group's website at ewg.org for up-to-date information on toxins in food and elsewhere in our lives. They have several handy apps to help you make good, informed shopping decisions. Another great resource for finding out what's in and on your food is www.whatsonmyfood.org

Every time you purchase an organic product, your dollars vote.

There is no question that fueling your body with good food will only help you regain health and vitality. Your body needs nutrients to function, heal, and repair damage—and if it doesn't get what it needs, you will remain in a state of disease. The trifecta of health—clean air, clean water, and clean, nutrient rich food—will act to both stabilize your environment through the reduction of toxin intake, and give your body the elements required to function as designed. You will feel better because your load is lighter, and believe me, you're going to look better when you are only carrying quality food in your pack. With clean air, water, and food now part of your gear, there is one last area where you can stabilize your body and environment—your personal care products.

Patient Story

Black Widow Spider Bite

I was set to leave on a road trip with my family for Thanksgiving, but the morning we were to leave I woke up and had Pink Eye in both eyes. They felt like they were on fire, but we hit the road anyway. After traveling for many hours, we stopped for the night and when I woke up the next day, I still had Pink Eye, I was also now in pain, and I felt almost paralyzed. It was the oddest sensation and it kept getting worse. I noticed a red mark on my arm and I began to suspect I may have been bitten by a Black Widow spider.

Despite my new symptoms, we drove for another 7 hours to arrive at our destination. I went straight to bed. When I woke up the next day I was in even more pain, and started to get scared. My jaw was tight, I was in pain, and my entire body was swollen. The skin on my arms and legs was so tight I couldn't even pinch it.

I called the emergency room and the nurse said it sounded like I had tetanus, or I had been bitten by a Black Widow. They suggested I come in and get a tetanus shot, but I wasn't about to inject more toxins into my body, so I called Doc Nuzum.

When I described what was going on, he agreed it could be tetanus, but more likely a Black Widow bite, especially since I had a huge red mark on my arm with streaks of red going out. I knew something was seriously wrong.

"Your body is under attack and we need to provide what it needs to fight back." Dan said. He asked me if I had any of his supplements and thankfully, I did. He told me to take a very high dose of Super Earth Energy right away—10 pills. That should make the swelling go down and relieve the symptoms. Then, he suggested taking 10 more at lunch, and 10 more at dinner. So, I did.

About 2 hours after the first 10 pills, the swelling in my arms reduced from the wrist down. I could actually pinch my skin and the tightness in my body started to fade. That was Thanksgiving Day. I took 20 more pills that day and followed the same plan the next day. By dinner time the second day, I was about 85 percent better—most of the swelling went away, as did the tightness in my jaw and overall pain.

I kept taking the pills and a few days later, all of my symptoms were gone. I experienced a drastic turnaround in about 2 days, thanks to Dan's probiotics (Super Earth Energy). I gave my body the support it needed to fight the attack successfully and I'm living proof that natural remedies really do work.

—Brian L.

CHAPTER 5

Toxins in Personal Products

Statistics show the daily regimen for men and women exposes them to toxic chemicals just from normal use of personal care and household products. Men, on average, are exposed to 85 chemicals and women, much more, at 200 to 500 chemicals. This shouldn't be too big of a deal though since the products that contain these chemicals are mostly applied externally such as cosmetics, lotions, perfumes, and deodorants, right? Sorry, but no. On average, we absorb 64 percent of the chemicals we put on our bodies, meaning our choice of personal care products is just as important as what we eat and drink. In fact, some studies show that chemical absorption through the skin may be more hazardous than if ingested because it gains access to the bloodstream directly, without being subjected to the body's normal lines of defense. So before you pack your favorite lotion and perfume for your hike, consider one more critical element of daily life where you can minimize toxin exposure and stabilize your body—your personal care.

TOXINS ABSORBED THROUGH SKIN

Your skin is a protective barrier that keeps the things inside your body inside, and the things outside your body outside. This is pretty obvious. It is also the largest organ in the human body and plays other important roles besides "barrier." Nerve endings in our skin communicate to the brain external conditions such as hot and cold. It helps regulate the body temperature through sweating, and even helps your body detox some types of toxins. The outer layer of skin completely replaces itself approximately every 35 days. Skin is pretty amazing really. But as good as skin is at being a barrier and protecting our body from outside harm, it is not impenetrable.

On average, it takes 26 seconds for a chemical to pass through the skin into the bloodstream. This of course assumes the chemical is capable of penetrating the skin—but the majority are able. Think about a nicotine patch or a medicated pain relief pad that you stick to your back. If our skin couldn't readily absorb chemicals like these, the nicotine patch would not be sold today.

The rate of chemical absorption in the skin is dependent on many factors. One factor is how thick the skin is, which can be roughly related to what part of your body is being considered. The outer part of your forearm has a much lower absorption rate than your forehead, which has a significantly lower absorption rate than genitalia. Increased body temperature also affects how your body absorbs chemicals. The warmer your skin, the more permeable it becomes. This is also true when it becomes wet, particularly when it is submerged for any period of time. Soaps and surfactants (the ingredient in shampoos that makes them sudsy) also neutralize some of the body's own protective chemicals, allowing a greater absorption rate. So, after a nice hot shower or long soaking bath where you have properly soaped up and washed your hair, your body is primed to absorb toxic chemicals from personal care products.

On average, it takes 26 seconds for a chemical to pass through the skin into the bloodstream.

Personal Care Products

From lipsticks to shampoos and lotions to toothpastes, there are thousands of different chemicals in personal care products. Only 20 percent of these chemicals have been tested by the US government for their long-term effects.

The European Union has banned over 1,300 chemicals from cosmetic manufacturing through Council Directive 76/768/EEC. The FDA, on the other hand, has only prohibited the use of 11 chemicals by name. This crazy statistic has been circulated around the internet for a while now, so why is there such a huge discrepancy between what the EU and the US think is allowable? The answer is available straight from the FDA website:

"FDA's legal authority over cosmetics is different from our authority over other products we regulate, such as drugs, biologics, and medical devices. Under the law, cosmetic products and ingredients do not need FDA premarket approval, with the exception of color additives."

So if the FDA doesn't have legal authority to make personal care products and cosmetics safe, then who is regulating them? Well, this is also spelled out on the FDA website:

"Companies and individuals who manufacture or market cosmetics have a legal responsibility to ensure the safety of their products. Neither the law nor FDA regulations require specific tests to demonstrate the safety of individual products or ingredients. The law also does not require cosmetic companies to share their safety information with FDA."

The cosmetic and personal care product industry is largely self-regulated. It's a good thing giant companies that specialize in personal care products would never jeopardize the safety of their customers just to make a profit (please insert extreme sarcasm when reading this sentence).

Of the 80,000 chemicals being used in personal care products, household products, and many other areas of the market, nearly all of them are inflammatory. The vast majority of them are known carcinogens, and in many cases, may be endocrine disruptors (chemicals that may interfere with the body's endocrine system). American companies produce cleaner, safer versions of many popular products. But due to differing regulations, the majority of these are sold to other countries who demand cleaner products. For example, over 11,000 unclean, or contaminated products, are banned in Australia, Japan, New Zealand, and all of Europe.

The US continues to sell its heavily contaminated products to Americans because they are allowed to. A major US company admitted to manufacturing and selling baby shampoo containing known carcinogens to US consumers, while at the same time manufacturing and selling a cleaner formula to European consumers to abide by their stricter laws and regulations. Interestingly, this cleaner formula is sold for a comparable price in Europe to the price of the unclean formula sold in the US.

Many chemicals used in personal care products contain carcinogenic properties or are active plasticizers, degreasers, pesticides, or harmful reproductive toxins. It is absolutely critical that you read the labels of your personal care products as carefully as you read the labels of your food.

The top 11 toxic chemicals or categories to beware of are listed below:

BHA and BHT

BHA and BHT are endocrine disruptors used as preservatives in many different cosmetic products. They are culprits of skin irritation and rashes, and organ, reproductive, and developmental toxicity. The European Union has refused to allow companies to manufacture and sell products that contain BHA and BHT.

Phthalates

Phthalates are another group of endocrine disruptors, widely used in body products. This chemical has been found to have negative effects on reproductive and neurological health. Phthalates are commonly listed as "fragrance" on the ingredient list of many different skin care items.

DEA (Diethanolamine), Cocamide DEA, and Lauramide DEA

DEA, Cocamide DEA, and Lauramide DEA are chemicals typically found in soaps and shampoos. Prolonged use in combination with nitrates creates a carcinogenic effect in the body.

Formaldehyde-Releasing Preservatives (FRP)

FRPs are preservatives used to prevent mold from growing in water-based home and body products and have carcinogenic and skin irritation effects. The amount of gas released is stronger in expired and old bottles of hair gel, shampoo, body wash, and nail polish. Use of FRPs has been banned in Japan and Sweden, and the EU has put heavy restrictions on their use. The following compounds are FRPs and commonly used in personal care products: quaternium-15, DMDM hydantoin, imidazolidinyl urea, diazolidinyl urea, polyoxymethylene urea, sodium hydroxymethylglycinate, 2-bromo-2-nitropropane-1, 3-diol (bromopol), and glyoxal.

Parabens

Parabens are compounds found in a variety of skin care products. In one small study, traces of five parabens were found in breast cancer tumors of 19 out of 20 women studied. If a product contains parabens, you will likely see one of these names on the label: methylparaben, ethylparaben, propylparaben, butylparaben, and isobutylparaben. Studies have found some form of parabens in the urine in up to 99 percent of people in the US. The EU banned parabens in 2012.

Dioxin

Dioxin is a compound found in lotions and deodorants, and interestingly, commonly found in animal products. Pregnant women are highly susceptible to dioxin's effects on the unborn child, and exposure can result in hormone dysfunction to the child.

Polyethylene Glycols (PEGs)

PEGs are chemicals most commonly found in body lotions and spray-on oven degreasers. Its use is to blend water with oil-based ingredients but is particularly harmful when applied to areas with broken skin and can cause an aging effect to the skin.

Petrolatum

Petroleum is a white jelly substance used to lock in the skin's moisture. It is found in name brand products such as Vaseline and Vicks VapoRub, and a variety of diaper rash creams. Petrolatum can be contaminated with polycyclic aromatic hydrocarbons (PAHs), which may be cancer-causing to humans, with a higher risk when left on the skin for long periods of time.

Siloxanes

Siloxanes are made of silicones. It is used in hair conditioners and body lotions. It is not water-soluble and will accumulate over time. There is little reported harm to the body, but it is very harmful to the environment, since it takes about 500 years to biodegrade.

Sodium Laureth Sulfate

Sodium laureth sulfate is a surfactant typically found in body soaps, creams, and lotions. It is what makes soap products foam and lather. It can cause irritation of the skin, eyes, and lungs. This is not to be confused with sodium *lauryl* sulfate, which has also been classified as a moderate hazard by the EWG.

Triclosan

Triclosan is an endocrine disruptor found in toothpastes, antibacterial soaps, deodorants, and shaving products. It has high levels of environmental toxicity by way of bioaccumulation and creates triclosan-resistant bacteria. It has been detected in the breast milk, urine, and serum of people and identified as an estrogen mimicker. Pregnant women and their unborn child(ren) are the most susceptible to the harmful effects of triclosan. Note that the FDA has stated that triclosan-containing OTC antibacterial soaps are no more effective than washing with soap and water.

For more information about the products in your own bathroom, visit ewg.org, a nonprofit organization dedicated to educating consumers. They have developed an app, called "Skin Deep," that allows you to simply scan the barcode of a product (or enter the product's name) to get an instant toxicity rating. It is a great tool to learn more about your personal care products.

Minimize Toxin Exposure from Personal Care Products

Take control over what you are putting on your precious skin. Protect yourself from long-term health effects by counteracting your exposure to these toxic chemicals. On a daily basis, use body care items that are rich in antioxidants like coffee sugar scrubs or pomegranate face wash. Using natural products like these help your skin build its own natural defense system.

Protect your skin from environmental hazards by wearing gloves when using any cleaning products, paints, and other chemical products that contain toxic chemicals.

Implement substances like fulvic acid compounds into your pill supplementation regimen. This keeps nutrients going in and the toxins going out of your cells. Tea tree oil has natural antimicrobial properties, and coconut oil is a natural alternative to lotions.

Choosing personal care items with organic, natural ingredients will drastically reduce the chemicals you are exposed to. Read labels on anything you purposefully put on your skin as carefully as you read food labels. Use EWG resources to help decipher the toxicity level of these ingredients so you can make well-informed decisions.

Remember, what you put on your body is just as significant as what you put in your body—including in your teeth.

DENTAL AMALGAMS

Many people still have amalgam fillings in their teeth that contain between 40 and 50 percent mercury. Amalgam fillings are often referred to as "silver" fillings, which is only a minor part of this material's composition. Once implanted into the teeth, mercury is not stable and constantly releases mercury vapor into the body, which continues to accumulate over time.

Mercury vapor off-gassing from dental amalgams is dangerous to the patient, hygienist, dentist, and the environment. The form of mercury in fillings is different from the increasing mercury contamination in the ocean and in many fish populations. It is elemental mercury that releases vapor and is absorbed through inhalation, not through our digestive tract as it is when we eat contaminated fish.

The greatest exposure to mercury vapor occurs during installation and removal of fillings, but vapors are also released when eating, clenching your teeth, or brushing. Heating up the amalgam also causes mercury vapors to release and can happen any time you eat soup or sip coffee or tea. Mercury starts to off-gas at 83 degrees Fahrenheit. The average human body temperature is 98.6 degrees Fahrenheit. Seventy percent of the mass of mercury amalgam can be lost in the first five years after it is placed in your mouth, and when mercury hits your stomach, the stomach acid creates a mercury delivery system. This is a big health problem that goes unseen. Elemental mercury damages everything it touches and it should not be something we should come in contact with.

I have rarely seen a patient with breast cancer, colon cancer, liver cancer, prostate cancer, or pancreatic cancer who didn't have mercury fillings.

I have seen very few cancer patients with any type of cancer who didn't have mercury fillings. Also, most people with thyroid issues have been exposed to mercury. In addition, mercury loves to bind to chlorine and to fluoride—they are best friends.

If you drink chlorinated water that contains fluoride, as the water passes over your mercury fillings, it is possible that small amounts of mercury are being extracted every time you drink. This can create compounds hundreds of times more toxic than mercury by itself because you are creating a delivery system for mercury to enter your body.

Research has shown through a series of autopsies that there were higher levels of mercury in the tissues of individuals who had amalgam fillings than in the tissues of those who did not have them. Mercury levels were higher in the liver, kidneys, reproductive organs, brain, saliva, blood, and breast milk of nursing mothers. Despite these findings, the American Dental Association has deemed it safe for use in dental offices and in your mouth.

Even small amounts of mercury vapor can be harmful to the human body. It can be inhaled and absorbed in the lungs and spread throughout the body via the bloodstream. It strongly affects the central nervous system—your body's operating system.

High levels of mercury in the body are associated with neurological damage, reproductive issues, and kidney failure. Some personal changes you may notice if you have amalgam fillings are fatigue, irritability, headaches, hand tremors, hearing loss, hallucinations, changes in behavior, and chronic pain. Globally, one in seven people are affected by chronic pain and it is often hard to pinpoint the source. Who would have thought it could be the result of your fillings?

Elemental mercury is a powerful irritant and is toxic to the body, causing inflammation and disrupting health.

The following list of afflictions can be caused by mercury vapor inhalation:

- Arthritis
- Fibromyalgia
- Parkinson's disease
- Alzheimer's disease
- Diabetes
- Depression
- Asthma
- Crohn's disease
- Candida
- Eczema
- Fatty liver disease
- Kidney disease
- Thyroid Dysfunction: (Hashimoto's, Hypo-, Hyper- Thyroidism)
- Reproductive issues
- MS
- Auto Immune Disease

Minimize Dental Mercury Exposure

Finding a dentist who will listen to your concerns is important. Most dentists are aware of the hazards of amalgams but still offer it to their patients as an inexpensive option. If your dentist attempts to convince you not to worry about the effects of amalgam, we suggest looking for a new, holistic dentist.

There is a safe way to remove mercury from your teeth. Be sure to ask your dentist how he or she performs this procedure because if it is done incorrectly, it can cause serious toxic exposure. I saw many patients that developed digestive disorders, kidney failure, thyroid disease, and systemic arthritis the following weeks after having their mercury amalgams removed improperly. Amalgams must be removed properly by an experienced biological or holistic dentist. For more information on safe amalgam removal, go to www.MillDental.com and watch the video at the bottom of the home page titled *Mercury Removal FAQ.*

My clinical protocol for people going through amalgam removal is to follow up with intravenous EDTA chelation therapy for 2-4 weeks after the procedure. Also, adding to this follow up, incorporate my Black Brew, Equalizer Fulvic Acid Spray, and Super Earth Energy for supplementation. Further still, complete a detox program every 3-6 months, or as required for your specific case.

RADIATION

Electromagnetic Fields

Electromagnetic fields, or EMFs, are produced by any object that uses electricity. EMFs can be electric fields or magnetic fields. Electric fields are created by anything that has voltage such as TVs, computers, outlets, and appliances. Magnetic fields are generated by electrical items with physical or electrical flow. The motor in your refrigerator is a good example, as is the electric meter on your house.

Any item that utilizes wireless technology also creates EMFs. Cell phones, laptops, Wi-Fi routers, cell towers, and SmartMeters are all products that create electric and magnetic fields and are a major source of EMFs.

EMFs are a type of radiation called non-ionizing radiation because the wavelengths are longer than that of what you might think of in an X-ray machine or nuclear radiation. In theory, these longer wavelengths are not capable of breaking molecular bonds, but that doesn't mean it doesn't affect the body—especially with constant exposure. The way it affects the body is similar to the way that nuclear radiation affects the body—it breaks it down.

If a wireless router can send Wi-Fi through the walls of your house, don't you think that same electric field can pass through your body? EMFs disrupt sleep patterns and hormones; they can induce similar brain patterns as seizures but without the physical aspects of a normal seizure. EMFs carry electrical information, and our bodies are designed to pick up information in very similar ways. We don't really know how disrupted our body's communication is because of this interference. What we do know is EMFs are increasing because we are all becoming more "connected," and our modern world depends on these technologies to operate. They are not going away, so we need to do our best to minimize them.

Minimize EMF Exposure

The easiest and cheapest way to mitigate EMF exposure is to put distance between you and the EMF source, or turn it off completely. Try not to sleep with your cell phone on the nightstand next to your head. Better yet, turn off your cell phone at night if you can to minimize the total EMF amount around you. If your home has a SmartMeter, chose a bedroom on the opposite side of the house to sleep in. And finally, turn off your Wi-Fi router while sleeping. Many people who have simply turned off their Wi-Fi at night have reported deeper, more solid sleep.

Radioactive Decay

Exposure to radioactive decay is less common but can occur in nuclear energy industry workplaces from large events such as Chernobyl to the recent Fukushima Daiichi disaster. These events can spread radiation contamination worldwide. Radon from the soil around your home is one source that often goes undetected.

The thyroid is particularly sensitive to radiation and many health issues can arise if the thyroid is compromised. If you know you have been exposed to radiation, add a quality iodine supplement to help protect your thyroid and overall organ health.

My supplement, Super Fulvic Iodine, is faster acting than other forms of iodine. It is much more bio available and is free of heavy metals, which is an issue in many other iodine products.

Personal care products, dental procedures, and EMFs are a major source of toxin exposure that we have a fair amount of control over. Choosing clean personal care products and making smart choices about dental procedures, as well as minimizing the EMFs in our houses, will assist our bodies in moving toward better health.

TOXINS IN VACCINES

Vaccines are technological feats, but many of their side effects can cause more harm than the diseases they are designed to prevent. Some simply view vaccines as another unnecessary exposure to toxic materials. Many parents are opting out of vaccinations altogether. Even the CDC website lists the following toxic ingredients in the vaccines that the pharmaceutical industry are producing:

- Aluminum
- Formaldehyde
- Monosodium glutamate
- Mercury
- Monkey kidney cells
- Genetically modified yeast (mold)
- Antibiotics (more mold)
- Pig and horse blood materials
- Chicken embryo cells
- Ammonium sulfate
- GMO soy and egg protein extracts
- Calf serum and blood materials

Vaccines are loaded with toxins. They contain heavy metals, animal proteins and cells, GMO products and the accompanying pesticides, including glyphosate, antibiotics, and additives. Some common vaccines, including those for chicken pox, hepatitis, and rabies, are propagated in cells originating from legally aborted human fetuses, according to the FDA. Vaccines can even predispose your children to many diseases, ultimately compromising the immune system they are designed to protect.

Most states still allow religious, medical, or philosophical exemptions to opt out of standard immunizations. Some states have eliminated the option for parents to opt out entirely, allowing only specified, government-approved agents to say if a medical exemption is justified. Parents are quickly losing the right to decide for their children what is safe and what isn't.

The topic of vaccinations is an entirely separate book, so I won't get deep into the topic here. Just realize they are a huge source of toxins for our children. There is a lot of research available for parents to read and watch, so they can make educated decisions. *The Truth About Vaccines* is a great documentary with incredible data on the subject. Visit www.thetruthaboutvaccines.com for more information.

EDUCATED AND STABLE

Each time we realize we don't have to cram something into our backpack for the long hike, we have a choice to lighten our load and stabilize our environment and bodies even further. Part 1 of this book was intended to educate you about the largest and most common sources of toxins in our air, water, food, and commonly used products. You should now understand how important it is that these elements be as clean as possible to support feeding the basic needs of your body.

My goal for you in this section is to take this knowledge and let it empower your decisions to reduce your toxin intake, support your health, and ultimately optimize your ability to heal. Keep in mind—implementing a few changes to your daily routine is better than not taking any action at all. But over time, work towards eliminating more and more toxin sources.

Step one of the healing process is to stabilize, and each time you implement another one of the solutions provided in Part 1, you are closer to being ready to move to step two, detoxification.

PART 2: DETOXIFY

Detox Concepts and Protocols

CHAPTER 6

How Toxins Affect Your Body

First, congratulations on your new education on how to stabilize your body by minimizing toxin intake. I think you will be amazed at how much better your body begins to function just by stabilizing. That said, if we stick with the overloaded backpack analogy, you may have already developed some issues because of the heavy choices you made to this point. It's okay. Remember in the introduction I said all bodies can heal, even when overwhelmed.

Detoxification is step two in the healing process, so Part 2 of this book will teach you how to properly assist your body to unload toxins. However, before learning how to lighten your pack through detox protocols, I want to give you just a little more education so you fully understand what is happening in your body because of the toxins. This chapter will discuss inflammation in great detail as this is common among everybody carrying a toxic load. The subsequent chapters explain more about what a detox is and things that happen in your body while doing a detox. Then, Chapter 9 covers how supplementation can assist your body during a detox. Finally, I provide four detox protocols to wrap up Part 2, so you can unload your pack and relieve some of the issues created to this point. But, before we get to the protocols, let's talk about some aches and pains.

YOUR BODY IS IRRITATED

Our bodies don't always tell us about the accumulation of excess toxins right away. It tries very hard to handle the elimination on its own, always thinking you are going to stop adding things to the pack so it can catch up. It becomes irritated with the situation and may even provide some hints that it's not happy. This is relative to the first couple miles on the trail, where you know your backpack is heavy, but you keep going because nothing is bothering you too bad yet. But, at about mile 5, you begin to realize how severely your knees are aching, your lower back is screaming not to go on, and you are getting a headache from the strain of the pack pulling on your shoulders. Your body has just signaled to you that if you don't change something soon, bad things will happen. It is no longer just irritated, now it is painfully inflamed.

All of these aches and pains are critical to realizing there is something wrong that you need to deal with. Yes, you can cover the pain temporarily with pain medication, but if you don't lighten the load of your pack, the pain will come back again and again. But why is pain often associated with the storage of toxins?

The Three I's

Inflammation is your body's natural defense system at work. It doesn't matter if it's an injury, stress, disease, toxins, or infection, the reaction is the same. Inflammation never just happens on its own. It is always triggered by some irritant and is your body's way of protecting the irritated area from further harm. For example, if you've ever experienced whiplash in a car accident, you may have noticed that you don't really feel the hurt until the next day. And you feel even worse on the third day. This is because the inflammatory processes are setting in.

The body deals with irritation first by adding water, which creates a wet environment. This wet environment causes swelling and reduces blood flow, and as a result will grow stagnant, making the body susceptible to infection. The three I's of disease development are always in progression: irritation leads to inflammation, and inflammation ultimately leads to infection. Understand the word infection is being used as a general term that could indicate disease of any sort, not just an actual infection.

Inflammation is an Impediment

Consider what would happen to a bucket of clean, distilled water that's been left on your front porch for two weeks. What would happen to the water? It would get stagnant and start to grow nasty bacteria and parasites. The same concept applies to your body. When joints or tissues are wet for too long, they become breeding grounds for infection. Your immune response kicks in, but its performance is less than optimal. Your white blood cells are trying to take ground, but they can't move very well in a murky environment. It is kind of like sending soldiers through a swamp and expecting them to fight as well as they do on dry land. They will still fight, but not nearly as efficiently because they aren't as mobile, and therefore, cannot stabilize the situation.

The communication network of your body is also impeded by inflammation. Your body has three different communications systems: nervous system, hormonal system, and an intracellular and extracellular system. You literally have a Wi-Fi system, where cells send electrical signals back and forth to each other. When tissues are normal and healthy, the cells are dry—they are closely packed together. They can easily communicate with each other and the Wi-Fi works well. But when tissues are inflamed, wet with extra fluid and swollen, the cells are farther apart and communication becomes more difficult. Signals get crossed and jumbled. Sometimes, they get lost altogether.

Temporary versus Chronic Inflammation

Inflammation is either temporary or chronic. Temporary inflammation occurs when an irritant invokes your body's normal, protective response. If you take care of the irritation, the inflammation goes away. Chronic inflammation also starts with irritation, but if the irritation is never addressed, the inflammation remains to protect the area. Think about a sprained ankle. If you stay off your feet and ice the ankle a few times per day, the irritated part of your ankle heals. Once the irritant is gone, the inflammation goes too. But, if you continue to jump around and run on your ankle, it remains irritated and the inflammation stays around much longer. As long as the irritation remains, the inflammation will remain.

At the onset, irritations can seem like a small thing and may be easily ignored, but don't ignore them. Your body is trying to tell you something. Irritation is the first of the three I's for a reason: it is critical to address early because if you don't, you're on a path to chronic inflammation. And chronic inflammation is the primary cause of serious illness and disease like leaky gut syndrome, inflammatory bowel disease (IBD), certain cancers, arthritis, heart disease, diabetes, high blood pressure, and asthma.

MOST DISEASE IS LINKED TO CHRONIC INFLAMMATION

Let's revert briefly to remind ourselves how seeking only the treatments of conventional medicine can easily derail us from figuring out the source of our inflammation. Conventional medicine typically focuses on treating your symptoms rather than finding the root cause of your health issues. Doctors ask what, rather than why. For example, they treat heart disease as an inflammation of the arteries, and arthritis as chronic inflammation in various joints. They prescribe pain relievers to relieve pain, diuretics to reduce swelling, and drugs to suppress inflammation, thus reducing the effectiveness of the immune system. In tandem, large pharmaceutical companies create drugs designed to treat the symptoms of this inflammation rather than the source.

Conventional medicine ignores the fact that just because it's possible to make the pain go away or the test result more favorable doesn't mean the disease is gone. The reason you developed the disease is still lurking. The chronic inflammation set the stage for "infection," but what about the irritant that started it all? Let's take a look at how toxins act as the irritant in many of the chronic diseases our population is currently plagued with.

Conventional medicine ignores the fact that just because it's possible to make the pain go away or the test result more favorable doesn't mean the disease is gone.

Toxins Cause Leaky Gut Syndrome

Irritation from toxins and food additives can cause inflammation of the semipermeable layer of cells that make up the wall of your gut. Toxins that are known to irritate your digestive tract include food additives, over-the-counter NSAIDS (non-steroidal anti-inflammatory drugs) such as ibuprofen, excessive alcohol, and refined sugars. Leaky gut syndrome is the condition where the semipermeable wall of your digestive tract becomes too permeable and allows toxins, undigested foods, and digestive debris to enter the bloodstream.

Under normal circumstances, foods enter the bloodstream after being digested and after the nutrients are already broken down. With leaky gut syndrome, undigested foods, toxins, and debris enter the bloodstream through breaches in the gut wall. When this happens, the bloodstream becomes overwhelmed.

Because the blood is essentially under attack from the toxins and debris, the immune system identifies these proteins and other components as threats and begins to produce antibodies to combat them. Since we continuously need to eat and the holes in the gut wall remain, the immune system quickly becomes overworked. This allows diseases to thrive, including autoimmune disease. Diseases typically faced by adults, like cardiovascular disease and diabetes, are now being developed within children.

In a culture like ours that thrives on busy schedules, our diets consist mostly of processed foods, designed for convenience and full of toxins. It is rare for children to eat anything green. Fresh fruits and vegetables are almost foreign to their taste buds. And so a cycle of poor health is created where one of the most common ramifications of a diet loaded with processed foods is leaky gut. And it simply stems from a significant lack in healthy food and nutrition, which also happens to be the remedy.

Now that you understand what leaky gut syndrome is and what causes it, let's look at some ways to avoid the problem. Treatments range from supplements, vitamins, and specific foods to simple diet and awareness. You can avoid leaky gut by eating fruits and vegetables that are rich in essential fatty acids and vitamin C. The most important thing is to avoid bombarding your digestive system with toxins, processed foods, undigested food, preservatives, and alcohol. When you avoid toxins, you give your digestive system the ability to work effectively and avoid a leaky gut. Another critical element to a healthy digestive system is your gut microorganisms.

TOXINS ALTER THE BALANCE OF YOUR BODY'S AEROBIC AND ANAEROBIC MICROORGANISMS

There are two types of microorganisms in your body: aerobic and anaerobic. Aerobic microbes need oxygen to breathe and are probiotic—they build up the body and are very beneficial. Anaerobic microbes do not need oxygen. They are the sugar-eating microbes that are there to break things down, to decompose things.

Aerobic Microorganisms

Aerobic microbes rebuild everything—all the way down to your DNA. These probiotics (literal meaning, *good life forms*) are loosely defined as live organisms that positively benefit the health of the host—you. These organisms are naturally occurring in your body but are also derived from external sources. According to the Mayo Clinic, "[probiotics] . . . help with digestion and offer protection from harmful bacteria, just as the existing 'good' bacteria in your body already do."

> You cannot achieve optimum health without probiotic microorganisms.

Anaerobic Microorganisms

Anaerobic microorganisms break down everything—all the waste your body produces from metabolism. If you eat a contaminated, toxic diet, this creates more damage and even more waste, which causes the clean-up crew to work even harder. You'll need more of these decomposing microbes to eventually eat through the waste, but this actually creates a problem. Since their only function is to decompose, they don't stop at waste. When they run out of waste, they start on you.

The Beneficial Microbial Balance

You should have more aerobic microbes than anaerobic microbes. If you don't do something to build up the good microbes, then the decomposing microbes will start to decompose everything—all the way down to your DNA. They start taking over.

Besides toxins, the balance of protein, fiber, fats, and carbohydrates in your diet also affect the microorganisms in your gut. Sugar consumption is a huge factor to the balance of your microbes. Anaerobic microbes love sugar and dairy. It is a key part of their diet to help them thrive, so too much sugar and dairy in your diet causes the reproduction and growth of anaerobic microbes, while starving the aerobic microbes. Additionally, the more the anaerobic microbes eat, the more waste they produce, which can create a toxic environment on its own.

Literally, how you eat, how you supplement, and what you drink will either feed one type of bacteria or the other. In order to feed the good bacteria, the probiotics, you need to eat foods that contain naturally occurring, insoluble fiber like apples, bananas, dandelion greens, artichokes, onions, oats, and flax seeds. These foods are all great sources of prebiotics.

The predominating microorganisms in your gut affect your food cravings, so if you have too many anaerobic microorganisms, you may find yourself craving sugar. Your diet can change the balance of organisms in your gut.

Often, your cravings are just a sign that your body is lacking in nutrients, either because anaerobic microbes are robbing your body of nutrients or your body is simply unable to absorb them because of toxin overload. The chart below shows what a typical craving indicates and how to remedy that craving with specific food.

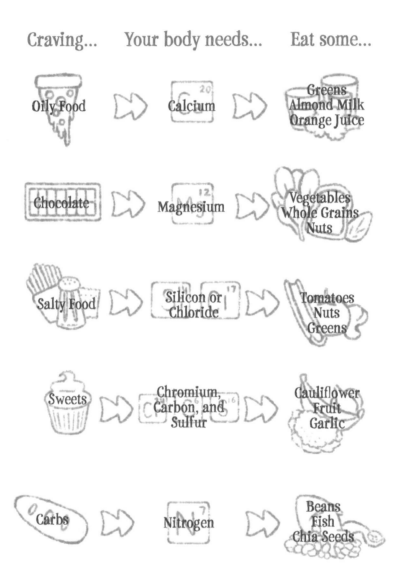

TOXINS CREATE AN ENVIRONMENT FOR CANCER

Cancer cells can be created by exposing cells to toxic materials, *or* by *not* exposing cells to nutrients. As we touched on in Chapter 1, heavy metals can enter a cell and block receptor sites from absorbing nutrients. This alters your body's normal processes and creates malfunctions in many systems. Malfunctions are also irritations that cause inflammation, and the cycle continues.

If you have inflammation in your body, you're wearing down your good (normal) cells. The more frequently your body must rebuild cells, the more nutrients it needs to function. If it doesn't have the right nutrients to rebuild the cells, it doesn't make good copies of them. We call these mutated cells cancer.

Your body is always producing cancer cells—cells that are missing some components of normal cells. All these cells do is eat and reproduce. Your body's immune system normally has the ability to stop cancer cells from growing, until it becomes too compromised dealing with chronic inflammation. Thus, chronic inflammation creates an environment that develops disease and cancer.

Cancer, arthritis, multiple sclerosis, fibromyalgia, cardiovascular disease, and virtually all chronic diseases are the result of the chronic inflammatory process.

The closer to the end of that inflammatory process you are, the more active the decomposing microbes in your body become and the faster you develop a disease you cannot survive. As long as the toxins are still there, the more inflamed your body becomes. But at any point in the process, you have the opportunity to change your body's environment, to begin detoxifying, and to decide to give your body the nutrients it needs by eating the right foods.

The Inflammatory Process and Cancer

We live in Idaho, home to beautiful mountains and pine trees. If we uproot a pine tree from Idaho and plant it on a beach in San Diego, that tree would never survive because the beach is the wrong environment for a pine tree. It needs mountains, it needs higher elevation, cooler temperatures, and it needs a specific type of soil—same outcome if we move a palm tree from a beach in San Diego and plant it in the mountains of Idaho. That tree wouldn't survive either because it's the completely wrong environment.

Applying this analogy to your body and cancer, we see that disease happens or grows because it's in the type of environment where it thrives. If you have cancer, it is because you have the right environment for cancer to develop. If you don't change that environment, cancer will continue to develop.

If you don't change the body's environment, it doesn't matter what you do to treat cancer. It will be futile because eventually it will always come back. The only way to heal your body is through detoxification. You cannot change your body's internal environment without detoxifying.

Not all cancer is caused by poor diet or chronic inflammation; it also depends on what you are exposed to. Certain chemicals can cause cancer almost immediately, almost on the spot, and can cause a significant amount of degeneration. Conventional cancer treatments including chemotherapy and radiation are universally toxic, referred to as cytotoxic therapy, or cellular poison therapy, because it destroys surrounding cells as well.

The only reason people survive chemotherapy is if they have enough good cells being reproduced to outrun the damage of the chemotherapy. The other problem with radiation is it can cause malfunctions in the reproduction of new cells, which can increase the chance of more mutated cells, or more cancer.

You cannot change your body's internal environment without detoxifying.

There is no question that our culture is overloaded with irritants. Toxins in our air, water, food, and personal care are constant sources of irritation for our body to deal with. The overburden of these irritants has caused an inflammation epidemic—we are sicker now than ever before. Hopefully now you can see how these irritants affect your body and lead to chronic inflammation, which leads to bigger problems and disease.

Addressing the source of inflammation is an essential part of healing disease. The next chapter will teach you more about detoxification as the essential tool to help your body rid itself of irritants. Where there are no irritants, there is no inflammation, and this creates an environment for health and vitality instead of stagnation and disease.

Patient Story

Rheumatoid Arthritis & Osteoarthritis

I was initially diagnosed with full blown rheumatoid arthritis in 2012. After many more tests and doctors' opinions, I was told I had both Rheumatoid arthritis and Osteoarthritis.

My symptoms were extreme swelling and sharp, burning, intense pains in the knees, ankles, hands, and elbows. Getting on an off the toilet or simply bending down to tie my shoes was a real chore.

Doctors put me on the following medications to try and ease my symptoms: Prednisone, Percocet, and Methotrexate.

I was taking methotrexate at the time, which gave my body a terrible reaction. I had kidney pain, vomiting, diarrhea, miserable headaches at the base of my skull, seizures that put me into a rigor mortis like state where I couldn't even move. It scared me so badly I quit cold turkey.

The side effects that lasted long after I quit taking the meds left me with urinary burning and complete loss of bladder control—I didn't even have a five second warning to get to a bathroom. I also ended up with esophagitis from all the vomiting and, twice, had to get tubes inserted into my throat to open it up because it was seizing up. In addition, my doctor confirmed sphincter damage between my stomach and esophagus due to the acid reflux and violent vomiting, leaving me with a hiatal hernia. In short, I went through hell.

I truly cannot believe anyone is allowed to sell drugs like these. In my opinion, it should be a crime.

It wasn't until I started taking Dr. Nuzum's products that my body began to actually heal. The inflammation and pain started going away in only 2 to 3 weeks on this combination. After approximately 2 months, I had no symptoms at all and forgot I was even diagnosed with any form of arthritis. Still, I was left with incredible damage to my bladder and esophagus and kidney pain to repair from the methotrexate. All of that is slowly healing now. If I hadn't experienced it firsthand, I wouldn't have thought it was possible to come this far in the period of time that I have.

I can hardly believe that in such a short time I could feel this good, compared to the daily hell that was my existence only a few short years ago. In addition to Dr. Nuzum's products, I also drink aloe vera juice daily as well as flax milk, and I have noticed further healing since adding healing whole foods to my supplement regimen.

At my most recent doctor's visit, all my labs checked out perfectly. I told my doctor that I'm healing well and happily without pharmaceuticals and will be staying on my current path. At that point, he asked what medication I was taking.

I told him I was only using plant based medicines and spoke about turmeric specifically. He said that he'd been hearing many good things about the healing power of plant based medicines and couldn't believe my medical history and that I'm healing despite taking no medications. He said as a general rule in the U.S., by the age of 50 most Americans are on five prescriptions and by 60, they are on six. According to his statistics and being 65 years old, I should be on six and a half pharmaceutical medications!

I thank God daily that I was led to these incredible, life-saving, health restoring supplements. I have my health back!

—Kraig K.

CHAPTER 7

Before You Detox

Detoxification is the second step in the healing process and a cornerstone of naturopathic and naprapathic medicine. It is a process over some period of time in which one abstains from, and rids the body of, unhealthy substances. It gives the body a break from the constant onslaught of new toxins and allows the body to receive good food and supplemental nutrition, enabling nutrients to fuel your cells as they are intended to do. And most important, this break allows your body to reduce the heavy load you are already carrying.

Detoxing the body is nothing new. It may be the oldest medical modality known to man, where various methods were used to cleanse the body, both spiritually and physically. It was a way of life that most cultures of the world followed. In fact, most indigenous medical traditions began their healing processes with detoxification, but for whatever reason our culture has veered from these traditions. How untimely, since the older our world gets, the more toxins increase.

I am confident you now have enough education about toxins that I don't need to convince you on the importance of detoxification. All of the chapters up to this point have emphasized this message. So as we move into learning how to detox, it is important to know how to properly prepare yourself for the protocol you choose to complete. Just like any big project, it is best to understand the goals, prepare your body, and make sure you have the materials required to succeed.

GOALS AND BENEFITS OF DETOXIFICATION

Understanding the goals of a project is beneficial prior to starting because it can help you prepare, both physically and mentally. Read through the following five goals so you know where you may need to provide additional support to your body to make your detox as successful as possible.

1. Clear Your Digestive System

A baby is a perfect example of a well-working digestion cycle. Shortly after babies eat, they poop. They eat again, then poop. As an adult, your body should do the same thing. However, because you absorb toxins and waste on a regular basis, your colon can become swollen with the accumulation and the cycle is impeded. Basically, your trash can is staying full instead of emptying on a regular basis.

Besides being your trash can, your colon is also where you absorb most of your water. When your digestive system is sluggish, water has to pass through waste that is not being eliminated in order to be absorbed. This continues a cycle of toxins being absorbed into your body, every hour of every day.

When your digestive system doesn't work right, a detox is your first step toward fixing it. Detoxification will help you improve your frequency of bowel movements and rebalance your gut microbe populations to support you, instead of inflame you.

2. Clear Your Skin and Lungs

When you sweat, you are detoxifying through your skin. You already know that when your primary detox organs are overloaded, the body stores toxins in your fat cells and lymphatic system. Sweating helps to remove the toxins your primary organs haven't gotten to yet. Think of it as an overflow system that you want to keep open to assist your other organs. If your skin is working hard to assist your other detox organs, you may develop some acne if the pores are clogged. As your other elimination channels open and become more efficient throughout your detox, this should clear up.

One great method to help keep your pores and sweat glands open is dry brushing the skin. Dry brushing is done with a coarse brush that removes dead skin. It activates the lymphatic system and removes surface dirt and environmental residues, allowing open channels to eliminate more toxins.

Your lungs are the first line of defense against toxins in the air and having adequate oxygen is key to detoxifying. Visualize your lungs as a cluster of grapes still on the stem. The main stem is the trachea. The large branching stems are the bronchi, the smaller stems are the bronchioles, and the individual grapes are the alveoli of the lungs. The alveoli are where you absorb oxygen and release carbon dioxide. Practice deep breathing meditation to open these alveoli to enrich them with fresh oxygen.

3. Cleanse Your Kidneys

Your kidneys work in partnership with your liver to filter toxins from your blood and eliminate them. Your kidneys filter 180 liters of blood on a daily basis. In fact, up to a third of your blood volume is injected into the kidneys with each heartbeat. They also clear your plasma up to 60 times, reabsorb water and ions, and secrete water.

During a detox protocol, supplementation is especially helpful to support the kidneys.

Vitamin C is extremely healing to the kidneys, as is parsley. The foods and supplements in our detox protocols will support your kidneys properly, but here are some additional foods and supplements that are particularly good for detoxifying the kidneys:

- Uva Ursi
- Burdock root
- Dandelion root
- Buchu
- Fennel seed
- Shavegrass
- Crushed watermelon seeds
- Asparagus

4. Support Your Gallbladder and Liver

Your gallbladder and liver are a large part of your natural, daily detoxifying system—your filtration system. The liver performs hundreds of functions in your body and is vital to several functions like digestion, detoxification, and more.

It produces bile which aids in digestion. It metabolizes carbohydrates, lipids, and proteins into material that your body can use. And in some cases, the liver also stores the minerals and vitamins found in these foods so that the body has a constant supply of the nutrients it needs.

You can support your liver and gallbladder by taking in supplements and foods that can help them in their processes. The juice of carrots and beets is highly beneficial. These juices help to flush out toxins from these vital organs by thinning the bile so that it flows freely, clearing the bile ducts of waste.

Additional support of the gallbladder and liver can be done with coffee enemas and herbal supplementation. One of my favorite liver cleansing herbal supplements is essiac tea—a combination of slippery elm bark, burdock root, shepherd's purse, and Turkish rhubarb. You can find more information on essiac tea, including how to make it, in Ty M. Bollinger's *The Truth About Cancer* (Hay House, Inc., October 25, 2016).

Herbs that detoxify the liver and gallbladder include:

- Milk thistle
- Turmeric root
- Ginger root
- Burdock root
- Dandelion root
- Artichoke

- Barberry
- Oregon grape root
- Chicory root

5. Lymphatic Drainage

The lymphatic system includes the thymus, lymph nodes, spleen, tonsils, and appendix. Lymphatic fluid (known as lymph) is a thixotropic fluid, meaning it becomes more fluid when warmed, disturbed, or shaken, then gels and hardens as it cools. Healthy thyroid and adrenal function maintains a healthy body temperature, which helps maintain a fluid lymphatic state so that it can properly flow and drain. This is one of the reasons anyone with chronic illness must achieve and maintain thyroid and adrenal gland health.

Spending time in a sauna is very helpful in detoxifying the lymphatic system. Just like butter hardens as it cools, so does the lymphatic fluid. Sauna therapy heats up the lymphatic fluid, liquefying it and freeing it so that it can flow easily. Using the sauna mimics what happens when you experience a fever; it enhances your white blood cell count and fights off infection and viruses. When detoxing, use the sauna for 10-20 minutes per day, or for as long as you feel comfortable. Do not exceed 30 minutes at one time or more than twice in a day.

PREPARE YOUR BODY

It is very beneficial to gradually prepare your body if you intend to complete a detox protocol. We recommend that you start by cleaning up your diet and your water for one month. You don't need to change the foods you are eating, but you do need to choose organic versions of those same foods. This may be an exaggerated example, but I use it to make my point: if you are eating cheese every night, continue eating cheese every night, but choose an organic version. Also, switch from drinking tap water to one of the filtered water methods discussed in chapter three. Remember, the first step is to stabilize before you detoxify by reducing or eliminating toxin exposure.

We also recommend incorporating some supplements to direct the process. (For this, we use Super Earth Energy, Equalizer, and Inflamagone.) Overall, preparing your body is very simple; switch to the less toxic versions of what you are eating and drinking, and add some supplements. This simple preparation is designed for beginners. It immediately eliminates a lot of toxin exposure by giving your body real food, the nuts and bolts that it needs to operate properly, and gently eases you into your first detox.

PREPARE YOUR PANTRY

Completing a detox protocol that lasts for a couple weeks can be a real challenge. One of the best recommendations we give our patients is to throw out the foods in your refrigerator and pantry that are processed and full of toxins and replace them with healthy, organic options that will support the detoxification process. It's way too easy to feel a little hungry and lose self-discipline briefly and snack on something bad. But if it's not there, you will choose something healthy instead.

Even if you don't throw away the foods that will tempt you, at least securely hide the following items until your detox is over:

Sugar

Sugar doesn't do anything for your body except appeal to your taste buds. It is difficult for your body to process, it crystallizes in your joints causing aches and pains, and it is what we refer to as "empty calories." Avoid processed sugars, especially white cane sugar, while you are detoxing. Natural sweeteners and those low on the glycemic index such as honey, raw maple syrup, coconut sugar, and stevia can be used in moderation.

Dried and canned fruit are higher in sugar than fresh fruit and should also be avoided. Fruit juice has very high amounts of natural sugar and some even have added sugar. Therefore, dried and canned fruits should be eliminated from your diet.

Proteins

Eliminate pork of all kinds, red meats, farmed fish, and canned meats. Avoid highly processed meats, soy products, and peanuts.

Canned Foods

Eliminate *all* canned vegetables and fruits. These contain toxins from the can linings.

Vegetables

Eliminate corn, soy, and potato products.

Fruits

Reduce dried fruits because they contain too much sugar.

Grains

Eliminate all grains, including wheat, buckwheat, bulgur, rice, oatmeal, rye, and products made from them—breads, pastas, cakes, cereal, etc. Grains and carbohydrates are the most complex foods for your body to break down. They cause spikes in blood sugar and when their energy is not used, the carbohydrates convert to sugar. Refined grains have caused many people to develop insulin resistance, high blood pressure, and heart attacks. Wheat and gluten overwork the liver and distress your digestive system. Eliminating grain-based carbohydrates will allow your digestive system time to rest and reset during your detox.

Beverages

Eliminate coffee, caffeinated products (except green tea), soda, and nut milks that contain carrageenan. There is more on this later so don't panic yet, coffee lovers!

Cooking oils

Eliminate vegetable oil, canola oil, safflower oil, and corn oil. Shortening should be eliminated from your diet entirely, both during and after your cleanse. These oils contain large amounts of omega-6 polyunsaturated fatty acids that are toxic to your body when eaten in excess.

Stimulants and processed foods

Detoxing is a great time to make not only temporary diet changes but lifestyle changes as well. I recommend cutting out coffee, alcohol, smoking, and other stimulants to renew your vitality for life and move forward into a new and healthy you. Prepackaged and processed foods typically contain high amounts of salt and incomprehensible ingredients that are toxic to your body. Commit to eating only whole, natural foods and eliminate processed foods from your home and diet now, and into the future. If it comes in a box with an ingredient list, you should not eat it. Specifically, avoid additives including MSG, maltodextrin, and carrageenan.

Processed chocolate

Eliminate processed chocolate products with sugar added.

Now that the above foods are gone, or at least properly secured, stock up on quality foods so you don't feel like your fridge or pantry is empty. Also, preparing many snacks and shopping for the meals you know you will make during your detox is key to being successful. Your body will be dealing with enough while detoxing, so even removing the burden of deciding what's for dinner will help.

Detoxing is not synonymous with fasting. We advocate using food as medicine to help your body heal and use its natural biological processes, working from the inside out. When selecting your detox foods, choose fresh, organic items that are locally sourced, when possible. Add the following items to your shopping list to be prepared for your detox:

Protein

Acceptable animal proteins are organic, free-range chicken, turkey and wild-caught salmon. Legumes, seeds, nuts, and quinoa are all excellent sources of vegetable protein while detoxifying your body. Limit protein to four to six ounces, three times a day, and make sure some of that protein is from vegetarian sources.

Limited Dairy

A limited amount of dairy and cheese is acceptable while on our detox programs. Raw and unpasteurized are best because they have active enzymes that will not clog the liver, as pasteurized dairy products do. If you are a cheese addict, you can have raw mozzarella, cottage cheese, or goat cheese every three days, but limit it to two to three tablespoons per meal. If you are dealing with a chronic illness or inflammation, we advise avoiding dairy completely.

Go Green

You are not limited when it comes to green foods. Include large amounts of broccoli, spinach, celery, sprouts, cucumbers, kale, and green beans. Green foods are rich in chlorophyll, which works with the body to eliminate chemical toxins, pesticides, herbicides, and heavy metals.

Colors of the Rainbow

Any and all vegetables are excellent. When you sit down to a meal, the more variety in color on your plate, the better. We recommend that 60 percent of your meals are vegetables and of that, 50 percent should be eaten raw. Our favorites are broccoli sprouts, asparagus, artichokes, and beets, because of their powerful detoxifying properties. Proteins and fruits should each make up 20 percent of your plate.

Some people with damaged digestive systems struggle when eating vegetables raw—especially cruciferous and leafy vegetables. This discomfort occurs because there is a lack of enzymes in the gut, which help break down fiber in these vegetables. Assist your digestive system by lightly steaming any vegetables that cause discomfort when eaten raw.

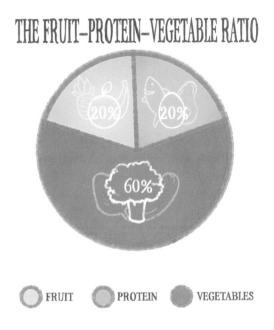

THE FRUIT–PROTEIN–VEGETABLE RATIO

FRUIT • PROTEIN • VEGETABLES

Cooking Oils

For cooking at higher temperatures, opt for avocado oil, which has a smoking point of 520 degrees Fahrenheit. For medium temperatures, coconut oil can be used up to 350 degrees. When making salad dressings and for use on cold items, integrate olive, almond, and grapeseed oils into your diet. Adding variety allows you to get the benefits of healthy fats and minerals that each of these oils can offer to your body.

Flavor Enhancers

All herbs and spices are welcome on your detox journey for vitality for life. Just because you are actively detoxing your body doesn't mean your food should lack flavor. However, do avoid seasonings that have added salt, MSG, or sugar.

Add fresh herbs to your meals and smoothies. Parsley and cilantro are powerful additions to any meal and aid in detoxifying the body of heavy metals, chemical waste, and toxic buildup in the kidneys. Consider adding a windowsill herb garden for ease of access to fresh, delicious herbs year-round.

Enjoy cooking with bountiful amounts of garlic and onions. Their sulfur compounds enhance the liver's detoxification pathways and are antimicrobial in nature. Garlic and onions are incredible for adding flavor to your meals without adding many calories and aid in killing viruses and bacteria that may exist in your gut.

It is important to note that if you suffer from acid reflux or frequent heartburn, large amounts of garlic and onions may trigger a reaction. If you experience discomfort, avoid using garlic and onions for the first part of your detox until your body has had a chance to begin its healing process.

Coffee

Yes, coffee was listed in the items to hide while on your detox, but for some this may be asking a bit too much. I would rather you successfully complete *most* of a detox, rather than fail because your body is addicted to caffeine.

Coffee raises your cortisol and it's a diuretic. For every one cup of coffee, you must drink three cups of water to rehydrate your body. Also, coffee is a stimulant that causes stress on the adrenal glands. These glands sit on top of your kidneys and enable your body to handle stress. So when you are under a lot of stress, like during a detox, your adrenal glands are already being pushed. Adding coffee is an extra stressor, which can lead to adrenal crashing and become adrenal fatigue—a common condition in America.

If you absolutely cannot give up coffee for the duration of the detox, reduce your coffee quantity and increase your coffee quality by choosing beans that are organic, fair trade, and non-GMO. Don't drink more than two cups of coffee a day and don't forget to increase your water consumption to balance the diuretic effects.

Detox Teas

Ginger, dandelion, fenugreek, green tea, rooibos, milk thistle, chicory, pau de arco, and slippery elm are all excellent teas for detox enjoyment.

Drinking these teas on a regular basis will help reduce inflammation and detox your body.

Proteins and fruits should each make up 20 percent of your meals. Vegetables should be 60 percent of your meals, and half of those vegetables should be eaten raw.

Each detox protocol you complete brings your body forward in the healing process and closer to optimal health. We want you to be successful in breaking the cycle of irritation and inflammation by helping your body detoxify in a safe and beneficial way. Preparation in advance is critical to that success.

Commit to memory the goals outlining your body's systems that may need detox support. Learn which foods to avoid and which to add to your diet, as described in this chapter. If you don't have to reference this book while in the grocery store, your chances improve that you will not only eat clean food on your detox, but will start to incorporate better habits as a lifestyle.

We also want you to know the background on detoxification so you aren't just going through motions. Rather, you are understanding what is happening during the process. Some of this was touched on lightly when we covered the five goals and benefits of detoxification, but there are other aspects you should be aware of before starting a protocol. The next chapter will explain more fully what is happening in your body, as well as some possible unpleasant symptoms you may experience during the detox process.

Patient Story

Breast Cancer

Just before turning 46, I was given the news by my oncologist that I had breast cancer. The news devastated not only me, but also my loved ones and all those surrounding me.

I lost no hope.

Because I had been under osteopathic care from Dr. Daniel Nuzum prior to being diagnosed, I put my life in his hands and he immediately put me on a special treatment. The treatment was a special diet which consisted of juicing, no sugar intake, and taking supplements such as Super Earth Energy, Inflamagone, Equalizer Concentrate, and his medicinal mushroom formulas.

Two weeks after starting the treatment, on my birthday, I was scheduled for a lumpectomy. The surgeon was extremely surprised because the mass he extracted was much smaller than seen on the test results. I was also shocked to see the amazing results in such a short period of time; it was a great birthday present to hear that!

The surgeon and my Oncologist said it was inexplicable and a miracle. I just said "the miracle has a name, Dr. Daniel Nuzum." Right after, I did the 2-Week Detox program. I purchased and installed a water filtration system and have been, for five years, faithfully following my special diet and taking Dr. Nuzum's supplements.

Thank you Dr. Nuzum for continuing to provide me the most precious gift of all—a healthy life.

—Odet C.

CHAPTER 8

Side Effects of Detoxing

Your body has been accommodating toxins, storing them in your backpack, and you have learned to live with them weighing you down. You may have even forgotten what it's like to *not* have chronic issues. Sometimes, it is only when you take the pack off and feel relief that you remember how you are supposed to feel. There are times, however, especially if you have never detoxed before, when relieving the toxic load can create some temporary challenges.

During a detox, changes start taking place in your nervous system, metabolism, microbial population, and even in your emotions. You may experience a variety of symptoms from the detox. Some are good and some may not feel so great. This is normal, but it's always best to be prepared. Knowing what to expect on your detox journey will further empower you and prepare you to succeed.

> Knowing what to expect on your detox journey will further empower you and prepare you to succeed.

EFFECTS ON YOUR NERVOUS SYSTEM

The nervous system is your body's monitoring and feedback system. It alerts your brain of any changes, good or bad, that occur in your body. It is also very aware of inflammation in your tissues caused by toxins.

When you have tissue that's inflamed, the swelling puts pressure on your nerves which the nervous system interprets as stress. Even if you don't feel "stressed out," your internal stress can be extremely high. The nervous system recognizes this stress as detrimental—or dangerous—which can activate your sympathetic nervous system. The sympathetic nervous system responds to dangerous threats and is more commonly known as the fight-or-flight response.

You are not aware of this directly, but your body automatically responds in several ways to deal with a perceived threat by:

- Inhibiting normal digestive functions
- Increasing heart rate and contraction
- Dilating blood vessels in muscles and constricting them in gastrointestinal organs
- Increasing sweating
- Shutting down libido

When your body is in a chronic state of fight-or-flight and your sympathetic nervous system never gets a break, you can easily develop stress-related symptoms, even if you are otherwise leading a relatively stress-free life.

Because we are not taught about this internal stress, or how to recognize when our bodies aren't functioning properly, we go on living with it. The internal tension comes out as anxiety, depression, ADD, and ADHD in children, and brain fog in adults.

Brain fog can happen when your brain and nervous system are overwhelmed from receiving massive inflammation feedback, and begin to bog down. It is similar to running too many programs at once on your computer, it has trouble keeping up.

When you reduce inflammation through detoxifying your tissues, you also slow down the distress messages from your nervous system to your brain. The stress is reduced and the sympathetic nervous system can finally have a rest, allowing the parasympathetic nervous system to take over.

The parasympathetic nervous system is the compliment to the sympathetic system. It is enabled or activated when stress and anxiety are removed. The parasympathetic system stimulates the "rest-and-digest" or "feed-and-breed" response. This increases salivation, digestion, urination, defecation, and sexual arousal—all those things you cannot do in fight-or-flight mode. Detoxification allows your nervous system to hit the reset button and may free up some emotions along with the toxins.

EFFECTS ON YOUR EMOTIONS

As you open your body's pathways by freeing them of toxins and harmful substances, it is possible to release memories and thoughts that may have been stored in the tissues as well. This resurfacing of past memories and feelings may cause you to feel un-characteristically emotional. Try your best to not become overwhelmed when you feel sudden anger, or the need to burst into tears. Just as your physical body is attempting to balance itself to a state of normalcy, so is your brain.

If you have some emotions that you have yet to deal with, such as resentment in a relationship or sorrow over the loss of a loved one, this may be a time to revisit and work through them.

Five Ways to Work Through Emotions during Your Detox

1. **Feel your feelings:** It might sound like advice that you would offer your five-year-old child, but feeling validated in your frustration and tears is sometimes all you need to release those feelings. Whatever emotions arise, embrace them, recognize them, and then let them wash over you before releasing them.

2. **Evaluate:** If you are feeling particularly angry or sad, try to dissect why. Finding the root of the issue can be helpful in moving the emotion forward to a resolution. Are you frustrated because you have created an unhealthy habit that is hard to break? Are you missing a pet that you've lost and are still harnessing that emotional grief? Sometimes, shining a light on the problem is all you need to scare it away.

3. **Find support and share:** Talking out some confusing emotions can be very helpful in the healing process. A number of support groups for a myriad of common issues are available in most cities and online. Confiding in a loved one or friend can be just as helpful, but may be met with bias or conflicting viewpoints. Support groups, therapists, and counselors offer a safe and confidential space to process your thoughts and feelings without bias.

4. **Avoid further emotional turmoil:** Detoxing your body is done with intention and purpose. Detoxing can be applied to other areas of your life as well. Remove toxic people from your life that may be causing you emotional harm. Avoid engaging in dramatic situations that may promote more emotional strife. Take a break from social media, the news, and current events to stabilize your emotional toxic intake.

5. **Be proactive:** Engage in activities that will help you process your emotional detox such as meditation and yoga. Taking time to be introspective is important during this time of renewal and cleansing. Various yoga poses can open your chest and joints where toxins and toxic emotions tend to reside.

Trauma and feelings can be stored in your body just like other toxins, and random situations can trigger them. As your soul tries to find resolution of toxic emotions, be sensitive to this and allow space in your life to experience the feelings that come up so that you can move past them. Forgiveness may be necessary, as well as grace for yourself and those around you. By taking the initiative to help yourself heal from past emotional strife, you are taking steps to a more emotionally secure future. One great resource is the book *Feelings Buried Alive Never Die*, by Karol Truman.

EFFECTS ON METABOLISM

You learned earlier that toxicity causes disruption in your metabolism by blocking the absorption of nutrients necessary for the body. Metabolism also slows down in an inflamed, swollen body because cellular communication is impeded by the excess fluid. Remember the foot soldiers in the swamp? Everything is slower and it's hard to lose weight in this state.

Detoxing has a side effect of stimulating all of your metabolic processes. When your body recognizes how much waste it needs to eliminate, it amps up your metabolism to handle the load. This can cause you to lose girth by getting rid of the swelling and the extra stimulation can help you better metabolize the food you are eating, making weight-loss an added possibility.

You must shift your metabolism into the anabolic (regenerating) mode from the catabolic (breaking down) mode to optimize your detox process. This shift is best stimulated through light exercise—it is the bridge your body needs to shift into that mode. Walking or rebounding on a mini-trampoline is a good way to help move your metabolism into the anabolic mode.

All of your metabolic processes are stimulated by detoxing.

EFFECTS ON GUT MICROBES

Remember the earlier discussion about two crews of microbes in your digestive system: anaerobic and aerobic? Detoxification removes the food source for the anaerobic microbes, causing a huge reduction in their numbers. The aerobic microbes will actually eat the anaerobic microbes as they die off, allowing more space for the good microbes to continue to multiply.

You may notice extra bloating or flatulence during this shift because, as the anaerobic microbes die, they putrefy and produce gas. This is part of the restoration of microbial balance and is totally normal.

You may also notice a change in your food cravings. The primary food source for the anaerobic microbes is sugar, which causes you to have a serious sweet tooth. Aerobic microbes rely on fruits and vegetables as their dominant source of nourishment and so will you, once they become dominant. This change in cravings usually happens the second or third time you do a detox, so don't be discouraged if you still want something sweet at first.

UNPLEASANT EFFECTS THAT MAY OCCUR

It is possible, and actually common, that the release of toxins from your tissues can cause some unpleasant side effects. This typically happens when elimination channels are not open and the toxins "float around" in your system before exiting right away. These issues can cause some people to give up on the detox because they think it is making them sick, but quitting early only forces the toxins to find a new home in your body instead of exiting as you intended.

The best method for minimizing unpleasant symptoms is to start with a gentle, or beginner, detox. If you jump into advanced detox protocols when your body is not ready—when some of your elimination pathways are not yet cleared and flowing properly—the symptoms can be quite difficult to tolerate.

Awareness and education are key to dealing with these issues, so here is a list of possible side effects:

Headaches

Headaches are one of the most common side effects people encounter during detoxification.

This is most often caused by caffeine withdrawal, if you are a coffee or "energy" beverage drinker. Try to substitute coffee with green tea so you aren't eliminating caffeine totally. It has a much lower caffeine content, but it may be enough to help with this symptom.

If you have chronic sinus issues, you may have a sinus headache or congestion during a detox. The mucus membranes in your ears, nose, throat, bronchioles (lungs), stomach, and intestines are actually all one continuous membrane. As one part detoxifies, so does the rest.

Hormonal fluctuations can also happen during a detox because you are eliminating hormone-disrupting toxins. Your hormones have to find a new level, a new equilibrium, and that can cause headaches in some people.

Changes in diet can also cause headaches. If someone is used to having a lot of sugar in their diet and they switch to having very little, they could experience mild to moderate hypoglycemia issues, which may result in headaches.

Nausea

Nausea sometimes happens during a detox protocol. This may be because of diet change when you transition from food that has very few active enzymes to living food that has a lot of enzymes. These active enzymes stimulate the liver and gall bladder, which can irritate the stomach and make you nauseous. Also understand that your digestive microbes are changing. The good bugs are being fed and the bad bugs are dying. These are events your body isn't used to and you may feel uncomfortable.

While nausea is fairly common, you should not be so sick that you actually vomit. This only happened one time in 20 years to one of my patients, and I found out later she actually had food poisoning.

Ginger and peppermint are both effective for minimizing nausea, as well as peppermint tea and ginger tea. Eating more apples, resting, and taking a bath with Epsom salts, baking soda, and essential oils may help. The very first time you do a detox can be uncomfortable, but hang in there. It will get better.

Constipation

Changing your diet may cause you to become constipated, especially if you don't drink enough water to process the additional fiber you will be eating. If you are feeling constipated, be sure to keep hydrated.

Eating apples and drinking chamomile or other herbal teas throughout the day can help a lot. One great herbal tea for constipation is Smooth Move by Traditional Medicinals, which can be found in most stores that carry organic teas.

Magnesium in almost any form can also help. Epsom salt is the least expensive and the most "moving" of the magnesiums you can use. Finally, you can increase the dose of Digestive Detox (my supplement for detoxing), do a coffee enema, or drink prune juice.

Hemorrhoids

Hemorrhoids can develop with straining or increased bowel movements. The irritation can be eased with Epsom salt baths with witch hazel extract. If you don't have witch hazel extract, the Epsom salt in your bath will still provide relief on its own.

Gas or Digestive Discomfort

When bad microbes begin to die, putrefy, and create gas, you may feel bloated and flatulent. Chamomile is very effective for relieving this discomfort. Equalizer Concentrate, our fulvic acid-containing product, enables the body to better deal with the beneficial changes in microbial populations that will happen.

Acne

Your body will store excess toxins it can't eliminate in the lymphatic system. As your lymphatic system starts to mobilize, some of those toxins can end up coming out through your skin, if they can't be processed through your liver and kidneys. You can develop skin rashes, acne, and boils. Try dry brushing the skin to remove dead skin cells and keep the pores and pathways open. As your primary elimination channels open and become more efficient throughout your detox, this should clear up.

Body odor

Simply put, body odor and halitosis can happen as toxins find exits through your skin and other tissues. You may have to bathe and brush a bit more often during a detox.

Yeast infections

Yeast infections can develop because of a change in your gut microbes. Taking a probiotic supplement, such as Dr. Nuzum's Ful-Biotic, may speed up the change from bad to good microbes in your gut, relieving this symptom.

Despite the many positive changes that will take place because of a detox, there are sometimes unexpected, or unpleasant side effects that can deter someone from completing a protocol. The effects of detoxification discussed in this chapter are not intended to discourage or scare you; rather, the discussion is meant to empower you with knowledge of what may happen and how you can minimize any unpleasant issues that should arise. Most of the time, simply knowing what is happening in your body (and why) will be enough to help you mentally power through a symptom.

> If you jump into advanced detox protocols when your body is not ready—when some of your elimination pathways are not yet cleared and flowing properly—the symptoms can be quite difficult to tolerate.

While willpower and education can take you a long way, it cannot make up for the fact that foods today are deficient in nutrients. Even organic, whole foods cannot fully restore some deficiencies in our body. Furthermore, asking your body to detoxify accumulated toxins demands even more nutrients that must come from somewhere. This is why I believe strongly that supplementation is critical for health and is the quickest way to fully support our organs and restore deficiencies.

Patient Story

Hashimoto's Disease, Anxiety & Depression

My name is Alyssa. I'm a wife and the mother of two incredible little girls. I have been struggling with thyroid and gut issues for more than half of my life. After a traumatic episode when I was fourteen, my gut decided it didn't want to work anymore. I was young and didn't know what was happening to me. I felt like I was constantly at the doctor's office asking for help and wanting answers, but they just told me I needed more fiber. On top of constant stomach aches and rarely being able to relieve my bowels, I was deeply depressed.

Throughout a span of four years, I had been prescribed three different anti-depressants, acid-reflux medication, thyroid hormones, ADD medication, and an antipsychotic by a stand-in doctor who had just met me five minutes prior. When they discovered my under-active thyroid, it was during an appointment to see if I had asthma; my thyroid was so swollen it was hard for me to breathe. By my second year into these medications, I actually attempted suicide. I cleaned my room, wrote my family a note, and took a large handful of one of my antidepressants, thinking I would go to sleep and never wake up. It thankfully didn't work, and it was obvious the medication I was on wasn't working either.

Over the course of fourteen years, I saw many different doctors in three different states, and none of them had answers besides more medication that only made me feel worse. In 2012, I felt that God started opening my eyes to food and how our bodies work; I could feel him changing my heart. I was once the girl who got irritated when she saw a "gluten-free" label! I thought it was ridiculous—that, and organic shirts and pillowcases. After I had my second daughter at the end of 2013, I really started falling apart. We had moved from Phoenix to Boise, Idaho, when she was only six weeks old (never do that, by the way…) and the stress of it all threw me over the edge. Something as little as the discovery of a spider near my children's toys would launch me into a full-blown anxiety attack that I couldn't seem to shake for an entire week and after that, it would take me two weeks to regain energy and strength. I felt like it would be better for my family if I were admitted into a ward of some kind! I lost patience so easily. I was either frazzled beyond belief or exhausted.

At the beginning of the year 2015, I decided to see how I felt on a gluten-free diet. Within two weeks, I noticed a tremendous change in my patience, joy, energy, and mental clarity. I decided I couldn't go back to gluten, and I also had a gut feeling that I wasn't done changing my diet. I went to my endocrinologist a few months later and told him of my new gluten-free diet. He congratulated me for feeling better but then said, "Changing your diet isn't going to make you feel better." That's when I knew that I needed to seek help outside of Western medicine. After that appointment, I got a phone call a couple weeks later from that doctor's office with my test results. "Hi Alyssa, so your thyroid levels look normal, and you tested positive for antibodies, so you have Hashimoto's disease." The woman on the phone said this so nonchalantly. She didn't know whether I knew what Hashimoto's disease was, and she didn't even ask me whether or not I knew. She didn't check if I was OK or ask me if I had any questions. I knew what Hashimoto's was, and it was the one thing I did not want. I was completely devastated and also shocked at how the person on the phone told me. Immediately after the phone call, I started researching Hashimoto's through the tears streaming down my face. I bought a grain-free cookbook by a woman who reversed her Hashimoto's through her diet and bought another woman's book about how she reversed her Hashimoto's. I could see the direction I needed to go, but I knew I couldn't do it alone.

I had heard of Dr. Nuzum from a few different people shortly after I moved to Boise, and I always had a feeling that I needed to see him. After that last appointment with my endocrinologist, who told me diet change would be useless and that he sees nothing wrong with diet soda, I decided to make an appointment with Dr. Nuzum. I was expecting to meet a man in his seventies because I had heard that he was so amazing, really knew what he was doing, and had deeply changed people's lives. I was shocked when I met him—not only was he NOT seventy, he was super buff and he has girls the same age as mine! How can such a young dude be so life-changing!? During my first appointment, I couldn't believe how much time he was giving me, and all of the different factors of my health he was looking at. I finally, for the first time ever, felt cared for by a doctor.

He was so encouraging and filled me with so much hope! He came up with a plan for me using supplements that he himself formulated and supplements from other sources he trusted. I left feeling more hopeful than I had in years. By my second appointment, not only was I walking into his office a different person, I felt the whole world needed to know about this doctor. There was a night-and-day difference in me, thanks to Dr. Nuzum and my diet change. I couldn't believe how quickly I was beginning to feel like my normal self again—my brain fog was lifting, I was steadily losing weight, I had more energy, and my face was looking like me again. There were moments when I felt it was too good to be true and I laughed to myself, "What did he put in these supplements!!?"

It wasn't long until I met Dr. Nuzum's wife, Gina and we talked for many hours. Both Gina and Dr. Nuzum know that I am dedicated to not only them, but I'm dedicated to helping other people get their lives back. I know what it's like to feel like years of your life have been lost due to poor health. I know what it's like to have such thick brain fog that you don't remember how you got home in your car or whether or not that stoplight was green after you drove through it. I know what it's like having no idea where to start with diet and lifestyle change. I am now committed to sharing my message of healing, just as I know with all my heart that Dr. Nuzum and Gina are committed to their patients.

—Alyssa C.

CHAPTER 9

Nutritional Supplements

The single most important thing you can do for your health and the optimal functioning of your body is eat nutritious, organic foods and drink pure water. This minimizes your exposure to most toxins and maximizes the nutrients so your body has the fuel it needs. Unfortunately, that is still not enough to fully equip your body to deal with the stresses regularly encountered. Stresses can be in the form of toxins, pathogens, disease, physical injury, demanding work, parenting, and emotional challenges in any aspect of your life. You need additional gear, even with a properly packed backpack. This is where supplements can help.

Supplements are defined as, "something that completes or makes an addition," according to the Merriam-Webster online dictionary. More specifically, we consider supplements to be vitamins, minerals, and botanicals that help your body rebuild stores of essential nutrients, assist in detox, and strengthen your immune system. They are an essential part of the detoxification and fortification steps in the healing process.

Some of the ways supplements help with detoxification are by:

- bringing a healthy balance to your digestive system and reducing toxic load
- supporting the colon and lymphatic system
- supporting the liver and kidneys
- improving nutrient transport and availability to your body
- trapping and removing heavy metals
- enhancing overall metabolism

> Supplements are an essential part of the detoxification and fortification steps in the healing process.

Because all of our detox protocols include some sort of supplementation, I feel it is important that you understand how they are benefiting your body during the process. I have listed some of my absolute favorite supplements individually, to help build your knowledge base. This information will also help you make the connection between the individual ingredients and the supplements we recommend during our protocols.

I do feel it is important to mention that my primary goal for you is health and vitality. Some readers may be offended that I mention my supplements, thinking I only care to make a profit by "pushing" them in this book. That couldn't be further from the truth. I mention them in this book because I have studied the healing properties of plants and natural medicine for over two decades, then developed some of the most viable supplements in the world to help your body detox and rebuild. I am providing the education on individual supplements in this chapter to give a better understanding of what I have formulated, but also so you can do your own research and make decisions for yourself about what botanicals you feel are the best for you. I want you to supplement your diet so your body can function at an optimal level, regardless of whether you use my products or wish to source your own. Please read the labels of any supplement carefully to ensure you are getting clean, organic, purely sourced ingredients. The most important thing to know is that no matter how good your diet is, you cannot get everything you need from food. You must supplement your diet.

THREE OF MY FAVORITE SUPPLEMENTS

Fulvic Acid

Fulvic acid is my go-to supplement for detox and nutrient supplementation. It is a naturally occurring humic substance that humans and plants need for nutrient assimilation, healthy cells, and detoxification. You can get it naturally by consuming plants grown in soil rich in humic substances, but that is very hard to find today due to industrial farming processes—so most people take it as a supplement.

One of the primary obstacles to supplement effectiveness and health is making nutrients available to your body and ensuring they are absorbed. Fulvic acid bonds to micronutrients and acts as a delivery system that helps the nutrients penetrate cell membranes, allowing vitamins and minerals to be absorbed by the cells and organs where they are needed. This is especially important during a detox because in order to efficiently get rid of toxins in your system, your body needs strength from good nutrition.

These are some of the benefits of fulvic acid:

- Enhances ATP (cellular energy) production
- Enhances nutrition
- Improves immune support

- Increases circulation
- Enhances detoxification
- Helps enzyme systems
- Balances hormones
- Stimulates metabolism
- Detoxifies, chelates, and neutralizes pollutants and toxins
- Enhances beneficial microbes

All of these benefits come from fulvic acid's natural ability to deliver nutrients where they're needed, while also removing harmful toxins. I describe fulvic acid as the body's mailman and garbage man rolled into one. As fulvic delivers beneficial compounds into a cell, it also picks up cellular waste and removes it from your system.

Fulvic acid is a critical part of my 2-Week and 21-Day Detox programs, and it can be a daily supplement for your detox lifestyle. You can find high quality, effective fulvic acid supplements at DrNuzum.com, including Equalizer Concentrate, Super Fulvic Iodine, Super Earth Energy, Inflamagone, and Black Brew.

Fulvic acid bonds to micronutrients and acts as a delivery system that helps the nutrients penetrate cell membranes, allowing vitamins and minerals to be absorbed by the cells and organs where they are needed.

Curcumin

Curcumin has health benefits for nearly every organ system in the body. It is found most readily in turmeric and is most widely researched and utilized as a natural anti-inflammatory substance. This orange pigment is a polyphenol, which means it's a vital micronutrient in your diet. Polyphenols are linked to health benefits such as cancer prevention, enhanced cardiovascular function, and brain health. By reducing inflammation in the body's systems, curcumin helps promote and maintain good health.

Curcumin is beneficial in other illnesses where inflammation plays a major role:

- Multiple sclerosis
- Epilepsy
- Allergies/asthma
- Rheumatoid arthritis
- Psoriasis

- Diabetes
- Obesity

Curcumin is a vital micronutrient, and must be considered part of a healthy diet.

Boswellia Serrata

I use Boswellia serrata in both oil and freeze dried form. This is one plant I love to use for helping my patients reduce inflammation, build their immune system, fight infections, combat leaky gut, and help with the healing of the hypothalamus gland.

When gum resin is extracted from the Boswellia serrata tree and refined, it is called frankincense oil, which has been used as a healing agent for thousands of years. It has gained much popularity recently in the aromatherapy world for its anti-inflammatory effects, immune system support and even cancer fighting abilities.

Numerous studies have proven that frankincense can boost your immune system by relieving inflammation in your digestive system. Make sure any frankincense oil you ingest is "food grade," as many oils produced are meant for topical application only.

In both oil and extract forms, Boswellia assists with swelling and inflammation. Clinically, it is used for inflammatory conditions such as arthritis and joint pain, autoimmune disorders (including lupus), digestive conditions (including IBS and Crohn's), as well as infections of virtually any kind. Adding frankincense oil or Boswellia extract to your regimen will go a long way toward a healthy and productive outcome. I use Boswellia extract in my Inflamagone and Frankincense Boswellia Serrata Oil formulations.

WHY I LOVE ADAPTOGENS

Adaptogens are botanicals that enable your body to adapt to stress. *Adapt* in this sense means to recognize and overcome. Stress comes in many forms: physical, emotional, chemical, nutritional, trauma, radioactive, infectious, structural, or psychological. And it doesn't matter what the source of the stress is, your body treats it the same— fight or flight.

In the last chapter, I discussed that the nervous system identifies inflammation as stress. It sends signals to the brain that there is a dangerous threat in your tissue, and your brain activates the sympathetic nervous system to deal with the threat. This system stays active until the threat has been neutralized. As long as the fight or flight mode is active in your body, you may experience reduced digestive functions, increased blood pressure, and reduced libido. If the inflammation is not eliminated, you can easily develop other stress-related symptoms, even when you don't feel stressed out.

The ability of your body to cope with stress, no matter the source, can be improved with adaptogens. These herbs have some of the most powerful antioxidant capacities of any source and are the most potent enhancers of your hormonal functions. Adaptogens enhance the functionality of your HPTA axis system (hypothalamus, pituitary, thyroid, and adrenal), balancing hormone production and overall, increasing your ability to cope with stress. They can even enable your body to withstand greater amounts of radioactivity, which is extremely important in the wake of the Fukushima disaster.

You are not restricted to taking adaptogens only during a detox, as most can be incorporated into your daily supplementation plan. Adaptogen sources include specific herbs, mushrooms, nutrients, bark, and roots.

Herbal Adaptogens

Amla Berry (*Phyllanthus Emblica*): High in catechins and flavonoids called gallates, this adaptogen enhances the effect of vitamin C. Amla is a neurological, immunological, and circulatory adaptogen.

Goji Berry (*Lycium Barbarum* or *Lycium Chinense*): Goji berries are similar to amla berries but are much higher in polysaccharides and carotenoids, especially zeaxanthin. Goji is a vascular, hepatic (liver), and renal (kidney) adaptogen.

Grape (*Vitis Vinifera*): Grape (skin, seed, and root) components are excellent sources of polyphenols, proanthocyanidins, and anthocyanidins. These ingredients are amazing anti-inflammatories and anticancer nutrients as well as powerful circulatory adaptogens.

Green Tea (*Camilla Sinensis*): Extremely abundant in polyphenols known as catechins, this amazing adaptogen is an anticancer, anti-inflammatory, and redox antioxidant adaptogen as well as an anti-infectious, neurologic, and metabolic adaptogen.

Hawthorn (*Crataegus Species*): Extremely high in flavonoids called oligomeric proanthocyanidins, hawthorn has been a well-known cardiovascular adaptogen for centuries.

Holy basil (*Ocimum Sanctum*): Its essential oil, triterpenoids, and phenylpropanoids make holy basil an amazing anti-inflammatory, oxidative stress, neurologic, hepatoprotective, radioprotective, cardiovascular, and immunologic adaptogen.

Damiana (*Turnera Species*): Given its diverse chemical mixture, damiana tends to be a neurologic, reproductive, sexual, hormonal, antioxidant, and protectant adaptogen.

Rosemary (*Rosmarinus Officinalis*): The carnosic acid, ursolic acid, and rosmarinic acid (all camphor-like volatile oils) make rosemary a powerful antioxidant, neurologic, and cardiovascular adaptogen.

Root Adaptogens

Fo-ti (aka *He Shou Wu, Polygonum Multiflorum*): These roots have an extremely wide range of phytochemicals and they collectively give *he shou wu* its vast adaptogenic abilities. These include neurologic, immunologic, cardiovascular, reproductive, liver, and kidney adaptogenic powers.

Rhodiola (*Rhodiola Rosea*): The rosavin, rosin, rosarin, salidroside, and tyrosol in rhodiola give it its powerful adaptogenic abilities. Rhodiola is an athletic, reproductive, cognitive, cardiovascular, sexual, radioprotective, chemoprotective, antimutagenic, anti-infectious, anticarcinogenic, thermoprotective, and hormonal adaptogen.

Ginger Root (*Zingiber Officinale*): Because of its phenolic compounds, sesquiterpenes and other components of the essential oil of ginger root, it has powerful cardiovascular, digestive, antioxidant, anti-infectious, pulmonary (lung), rheumatologic, and anti-neoplastic adaptogenic properties.

Turmeric (*Curcuma Longa*): Due to the various lipid-soluble phenolic curcuminoids in turmeric, its adaptogenic abilities are anti-inflammatory, anticarcinogenic, antimutagenic, radioprotective, cardiovascular, antioxidant, and antithrombotic (anti-clotting of the blood) adaptogen.

Suma (*Pfaffia Paniculate*): Due to its saponin content (particularly stigmasterol, sitosterol, and nortriterpenoids) along with its polyphenols, naturally occurring germanium content, not to mention suma's beta-ecdysterones, suma is an excellent hormonal, neurological, immunologic, cardiovascular, anti-inflammatory, antitumoral, and athletic adaptogen.

Eluthero (*Elutherococcus Senticosus*): Eluthero has multiple steroidal glycosides that give it its powerful adaptogenic capacity. Reportedly the most extensively researched of all adaptogens, eluthero—sometimes called Siberian ginseng—is beneficial in almost every situation that produces stress. The different adaptogenic effects of eluthero are antiviral, anabolic, antitoxic, immunoregulatory, chemoprotective, radioprotective, neurologic, gonadotrophic, and insulintrophic.

Nettle (*Urtica Dioica*): When I hear nettle root, I think urinary tract. Nettle root is an excellent renal, bladder, and prostatic adaptogen, whereas the nettle leaf is an excellent immunoadaptogen and sinus/ENT (ear, nose, and throat) adaptogen.

Astragalus Root (*Astragalus Membranaceus*): Astragalus is excellent for the immune system. The adaptogenic activity of astragalus comes from the polysaccharides in the root. Astragalus is a neurologic, protective, antiviral, anti-infectious, lymphatic, immunologic, immunomodulatory, chemoprotective, cardiovascular, and renal adaptogen.

Licorice Root (*Glycyrrhiza Glabra*): This triterpene and polyphenol-based adaptogen has amazing antiviral, antiulcer, antimicrobial, anti-inflammatory, anticancer, and cortisol adaptogen effects. Due to its ability to raise cortisol and aldosterone, it can also raise blood pressure. This is good for those with low blood pressure but not for those with high blood pressure.

Iporuru Root (*Alchornea Castaneifolia*): Iporuru is excellent for adapting to everyday wear and tear of the joints. This powerful root from the Amazon is the worst enemy of arthritis. Iporuru is a neurologic, fibrogenic, ligamentic, hormonal, and digestive adaptogen.

Bark Adaptogens

Catuaba (*Erythroxylum Catuaba*): The alkaloids, sesquiterpenes, flavonoids, and flavalignans give catuaba its powerful adaptogenic effects. It is an antiviral, anti-infectious, neurologic, cardiovascular, hormonal, and sexual adaptogen.

Muira Puama (*Ptychopetalum Olacoides*): Neuroprotective, androgenic, nootropic (used to enhance memory or cognitive functions), redox antioxidant, hormonal, and sexual adaptogen. This is due to the sesquiterpenes, monoterpenes, and alkaloids it contains.

Mucuna (*Mucuna Pruriens*): This amazing bean and pod from India is an adaptogenic powerhouse. By regulating dopamine and dopamine metabolism along with chymotrypsin and trypsin inhibitors, mucuna is a super power in the field of neurologic adaptogens. It serves as a neurologic, sexual, hormonal, and digestive adaptogen.

Chuchuhauasi (*Maytenus Ebenifolia*): As an adaptogen, chuchuhauasi is second to none as an anti-inflammatory and joint health adaptogen. It is an excellent neurologic, arthritic, anti-inflammatory, digestive, antitumoral, immunomodulator, hormonal, and sexual adaptogen. This is due to the triterpenes, sesquiterpenes, and flavanols it contains.

Mushroom Adaptogens

Cordyceps (*Cordyceps Sinensis*): Cordyceps is my favorite mushroom, and I have been taking it for over 20 years. It is a powerful antioxidant, immunoregulator, respiratory, liver, cardiovascular, kidney, sexual, hormonal, neurologic, radioprotective, chemoprotective, antitumoral, antiasthma, antisenescence (enhances memory), and athletic adaptogen. This is primarily due to both the polysaccharides and the D-mannitol that it produces.

Reishi (*Ganoderma Lucidum*): Excellent for immune support, reishi builds and rebuilds the immune system. The primary active ingredients are the polysaccharides and triterpenes. This adaptogen is amongst the most powerful of adaptogens and is a neuroprotectant, memory enhancer, cardiovascular, chemoprotective, radioprotective, hepatoprotective, renoprotective, hypotensive, immunomodulator, antitumoral adaptogen and even prevents altitude sickness.

Chaga (*Inonotus Obliquus*): Chaga is the most researched mushroom in history and is a powerful anti-inflammatory, antitumoral, anti-infectious, cytokines regulator, immunomodulator, digestive, dermatologic, antioxidant, and hepatic adaptogen. It has been determined that this medicinal powerhouse is antiviral, antimicrobial, and antitumoral, and it enhances both primary as well as secondary immunologic functions.

Turkey Tail (*Coriolus Versicolor*): Turkey tail has an enormous number of beta-glucan polysaccharides that heal the immune system and re-educate it. This makes turkey tail a powerful immune system, digestive, antiviral, anticancer, antitumoral, hepatoprotectant, renoprotectant, and neurologic adaptogen.

SUPPLEMENTS AS A PART OF YOUR DETOX LIFESTYLE

We have already discussed in depth how the standard American diet cannot supply adequate quantities of essential nutrients. As biological systems, we require materials to rebuild ourselves on every level, from our cells all the way out. You will experience metabolic dysfunction if you are nutrient deficient, but nutritional deficiency coupled with toxicity creates destructive metabolic dysfunction which can lead to obesity, diabetes, and immunodeficiency as well as autoimmunity.

Supplements are designed to supply what you're missing. You can expand and improve your diet, but because industrial farming practices over the last 150 years in the United States have stripped the soil of nutrients, the plants we eat do not have what we need—especially in terms of minerals. Because it takes nutrients for your body to perform the digestive processes on a nutritionally deficient food, you are in effect robbing Peter to pay Paul. The result is your body becomes even more nutrient deficient. You need a more concentrated source of what you are missing to make up for that lack. This is where supplements help you.

> Because it takes nutrients for your body to perform the digestive processes on a nutritionally deficient food, you are in effect robbing Peter to pay Paul.

Your body runs on enzymatic chemical reactions. The enzymes that control those reactions are each made up of a protein molecule and a mineral, such as magnesium or iron. If you're missing one of the components of the protein molecule or you're missing the mineral, you can't make the enzyme and these reactions cannot occur.

It takes 86 enzymatic reactions for your heart to beat one time. That is 86 different kinds of enzymes, each needing a mineral to function. Your liver has 65,000 enzymatic reactions that it performs about every three minutes. If your liver is missing selenium, your liver can't even clean itself out, let alone act as a filter for your body. Zinc-dependent enzymes repair all proteins in your body, including your skin and eyes. Everything in your body is made of protein. You can quickly grasp how being nutrient deficient can have grave consequences.

COMMON NUTRIENT DEFICIENCIES

Many Americans suffer, unknowingly, from one or more nutrient deficiencies. Older Americans are even more likely to be deficient because the body's ability to absorb some nutrients decreases with age. The four most common deficiencies within the US population are magnesium, vitamin D, vitamin B12, and vitamin A.

MAGNESIUM

Up to 80 percent of Americans are deficient in magnesium, and they have no idea. This is particularly worrisome when you review the common signs of the deficiency:

- High blood pressure
- Anxiety and depression
- Headaches and migraines
- Cardiac problems and irregular heartbeat
- Diabetes
- Chronic fatigue

Foods Rich in Magnesium

Dark, leafy, green vegetables like spinach, seaweed, and Swiss chard are the best food sources of magnesium. Other sources include beans, nuts, seeds, and avocado.

Supplemental Treatment

Fulvic acid supplements have shown a direct correlation with lowering blood pressure, when taken regularly. Lowering blood pressure also directly helps with other cardiac problems. Fulvic acid does this by adding magnesium to your system, making these dangerous magnesium deficiency problems a thing of the past.

Fulvic acid may even help you overcome your deficiency altogether, by improving your ability to absorb nutrients from your food.

VITAMIN D

If you struggle to get outdoors due to health, work, or some other factor, you most likely have a vitamin D deficiency. If you routinely wear sunscreen, you are preventing your body from absorbing vitamin D from the sun. It's difficult to get enough vitamin D from your diet—your body's natural process for obtaining it is from the sun's energy on your skin.

Vitamin D deficiency can become dangerous for individuals who:

- Are over the age of 50
- Have darker skin tone
- Struggle with obesity
- Have a history of depression
- Have a compromised immune system

Natural Source

The quickest way to treat vitamin D deficiency is with a moderate amount of sun exposure each day. You should also avoid processed foods with GMO ingredients, as they interfere with the enzymes responsible for activating the vitamin D in your body.

Supplemental Treatment

Another way to help counteract a vitamin D deficiency is by taking curcumin extract. This special extract not only helps reduce inflammation in your organs which prohibits the movement of vitamin D in the body, but is also key to promoting a healthy immune system and elevating mood. Curcumin is one of the most important adaptogens I rely on.

VITAMIN B12

Vitamin B12 is known as the energy vitamin. A deficiency in this vitamin results in a serious drop in quality of life. Here are just a few symptoms:

- Inability to concentrate
- Memory problems
- Mood swings
- Depression
- Constantly feeling tired
- Muscle weakness or twitches

Foods Rich in Vitamin B12

The best sources of vitamin B12 are animal products. However, those aren't an option for vegetarians and vegans. Even if you are a carnivore, most Americans need to eat less meat, not more. Taking a B12 supplement may be the safest way to eliminate this deficiency.

Supplemental Treatment

We also recommend our Super Fulvic Iodine supplement. This formula works quickly to support efficient metabolism and cell movement, so your body is ready take on the multitude of symptoms caused by a B12 deficiency. The fulvic acid in this compound can help improve efficiency of absorption as well.

VITAMIN A

You probably already know that vitamin A is great for your skin, teeth, and vision. Many people don't register, however, that a problem in these areas may be because of a deficiency. Just adding more foods rich in vitamin A may help fix problems like acne, increased cavities, and vision struggles, not to mention that vitamin A is an excellent antiviral.

Foods Rich in Vitamin A

- Grass-fed organic beef and poultry
- Colorful fruits and vegetables, like carrots

Supplemental Treatment

One of the first things people notice when they start taking fulvic acid supplements is the improvement in their hair, skin, and nails. Personally, I notice it in my skin and nails (I'm bald so I don't notice it in my hair, haha). Fulvic acid dramatically improves the problems brought on by vitamin A deficiency. This is because of fulvic acid's ability to help in the maintenance and regrowth of cells in these areas of your body.

Our fulvic acid complex has high concentrations of boron, calcium, copper, iron, magnesium, manganese, and zinc as well as other essential minerals. One of fulvic acid's most valuable features is its ability to repair salvageable nutrients and make them viable again, basically recycling these spent nutrients. If the nutrient is not salvageable, fulvic acid will absorb it and use its components to repair other tissues, cells, or nutrients.

> Be aware that botanicals can sometimes react in different ways with pharmaceuticals. If you are currently taking pharmaceutical medications, please consult with your medical doctor before taking any new supplements to be sure there will not be any negative reactions.

Supplements are designed to supply what we're missing. They provide a concentrated source of nutrients to make up for deficiencies, enhance your ability to deal with stress, and supply the building blocks your body needs for normal function. I firmly believe that proper supplementation is critical to health, during a detox and as part of your daily regimen. My hope is that you now have a better education about specific supplements and how they can support your body. Consider them the additional gear for your hike, that will make everything much easier.

I have used the first nine chapters of this book to give you a foundation of knowledge. This foundation is essential, in my opinion, to making detoxification part of your lifestyle. I do believe that knowledge is power, and that it gives us the ability to make educated decisions about the way we oxygenate, hydrate, fuel, and clean our bodies. It helps us recognize when our body may not be operating optimally and gives us the tools to assist our body to naturally restore health. Use everything you have learned to this point to decide which of the detox protocols in the next chapter is right for you.

Patient Story

Testimonial on Supplements

As a holistic health consultant, part of my work is finding supplements that are effective as well as consisting of clean, vital ingredients. Finding supplements that meet the needs of people with food allergies, heavy metal toxicity, or vaccine damage is one of my main priorities. Clean ingredients equal organic, non-GMO, dairy free, soy free, corn free, gluten-free and peanut-free. Finding companies that can accommodate this has proven to be quite difficult. Finding formulators that understand the requirements of not adding more toxins when you're trying to help somebody revitalize their health is incredibly important. I found that Dr. Nuzum and his line of formulations meet my optimal requirements. Not only has it been a great experience for my clients, but also for my family—including our dog, Brin. Brin tore her feet up on the ice and I tried every remedy that I could find, even making my own salves for her feet and booties. We tried for months with only minimal improvement. Thankfully, I tried Dr. Nuzum's Equalizer Concentrate and with daily spraying on her feet, the sores were dramatically reduced within a few days. After one week, her feet were completely clear of all sores and have remained healthy.

—Allie L.

CHAPTER 10

Detox Protocols

In this chapter, I finally get to introduce you to my detox protocols—the programs that I've created to fit the needs of anyone who is ready for the hike. All that you've learned up to this point has culminated in these practical applications. You may be excited and ready to implement all you've learned. Or, you may feel you're not ready emotionally, mentally, or physically to take this step. You may be examining your own views on toxins, whole foods, pure water, and supplements. These are perfectly acceptable places to be. With a spirit of learning and openness to new information, you're already on a better path. No matter where you're at emotionally, mentally, and physically, detoxing can only extend benefits of health.

It is my personal conviction that detoxification is a necessary part of health and for prevention of disease. Detoxing should be a normal, natural part of your life so you can take control of your health. Remember, at all times you are either moving toward health, or toward disease.

> Detoxification is very important to establish health. It is a long process. I will repeat this: because disease takes time to build, detoxing takes time to remove the contributing effects that brought on the disease.

There are three detox protocols in total:

1. 3-Day Liquid Detox
2. 2-Week Detox
3. 21-Day Detox

This is intended to give you flexibility in the amount of time required, intensity, and desired outcome. Read through each one carefully before deciding where to start.

Each protocol identifies who should do the detox, the benefits of the detox, specific foods and supplements, and daily instructions. You may have to refer back to chapter seven to refresh your memory on what foods are acceptable and which are to be avoided. You may also need to reference chapter seven if you have detox side effects.

The protocols are intended to be done separately, not at once. I am only saying this because we get asked all the time if people can "double up" on the protocols. Please just do one at a time.

Also, another very common question is whether or not the supplements are required. The short answer is no, they are not required. The appropriate answer is, if you want to maximize toxin elimination and optimize the rebuilding of your body, the supplements are pretty important.

Please do not start a detox protocol if you are pregnant or nursing.

And finally, please read through the following legal information:

The products listed in this material have not been evaluated by the United States Food and Drug Administration. They are not intended to diagnose, treat, cure, or prevent disease. You should not use this information for a diagnoses or treatment of any health problem or as a substitute for medication prescribed by your physician and/or health care provider. This information is for educational purposes only. You should consult with a physician or health care provider before starting any diet, exercise, or supplement program. Neither Dr. Nuzum nor his publisher are liable for any misunderstanding or misuse of information contained in these programs.

Detox
Protocols

3-DAY LIQUID DETOX

During this detox, as the name implies, you will consume only liquids to minimize the energy required by your digestive system, freeing it up to eliminate toxins. The workhorse of this detox protocol is fresh juices, but also allowed is vegetable broth and chamomile tea.

Juicing is very powerful and provides the body with concentrated phytonutrients. Phytonutrients are the sometimes-colorful, protective compounds made by plants. We call many of them antioxidants. The phytonutrients found in natural juices support the body's filtration system (the liver and kidneys) in cancer prevention and recovery from cancer treatment. Phytonutrients are also crucial for defense against autoimmune diseases, heavy metal toxicity, thyroid dysfunction, hormone imbalance, and vaccine injury. Finally, juicing is so beneficial because raw juices supply naturally occurring, live enzymes that add to your enzyme bank.

In addition to fresh juices, you should drink gut healing vegetable broth that will help repair some of the damage in your digestive system and provide additional nutrients. The warmth of the broth also helps trick your brain into thinking it's getting a warm meal. Hot chamomile tea is also allowed.

This detox protocol can be done over a weekend and includes a specific order of cleansing and detoxifying broth and juice formulas that you can make yourself. All of the recipes can be found in the final section of this book.

WHO SHOULD DO THIS DETOX

A 3-day liquid fast is for those who want to give their body a break from heavy foods and cleanse in a gentle way. Doing this every other month helps the body reduce daily toxic buildup and stimulates the body to release toxins and to open up detoxification pathways. This is also perfect if you need a quick reset and don't have two weeks or 21 days to do a full detox protocol. This 3-day liquid detox is not recommended for diabetics, pregnant or nursing women, children under the age of 12, or those who are in the midst of intense athletic training.

Juicing should be introduced gradually, particularly to those who are taking medication, are experiencing a health crisis, or have cancer. If you have never juiced before, take time to see how your body is reacting—listen to your body. You may feel tired, get headaches, and feel cranky or even dizzy at times. Don't plan on a busy schedule that will overextend you mentally or physically.

Warm, organic herbal teas are very soothing to the body and can help ease one through the detox process, especially when the person is having difficulty with the process.

LIQUIDS TO DRINK DURING THE 3-DAY LIQUID DETOX

- Cold-pressed juice, preferably made at home with organic ingredients
- Homemade, gut healing vegetable broth
- Chamomile tea

The broth and juices will help to keep your belly satisfied, however surviving on liquids alone may be quite hard if you haven't done it before. If this is your first time and you feel that you can't continue with just liquids, eat some of the cooked vegetables you will have left after making the veggie broth. Try not to exceed one cup per day.

TOOLS YOU WILL NEED

- Juicer
- Blender
- Stock pot for making veggie broth
- Room in your refrigerator for all your ingredients

FOODS TO AVOID DURING THE JUICE DETOX

Obviously, solid foods in general should be avoided for this short detox. If you are a coffee drinker, you should not drink coffee during this time. Be aware of the caffeine withdrawal discomfort you may experience such as headaches.

Substitute green tea for coffee if you experience caffeine withdrawals. The caffeine in green tea is more easily processed by your body and can ease a headache as it helps the liver and kidneys detoxify. I recommend that you begin to decrease your daily coffee amount two weeks before doing this for better results and also to feel better while juicing. Don't overthink—it is only three days and your health is worth it!

SUPPLEMENTS

The following supplements are optional but can enhance the detoxing effect you experience. Use as directed on the bottle for the three days of detox and continue on until the product is finished. You can find these at DrNuzum.com.

Super Earth Energy: This formula supports the adrenal and thyroid glands as well as the body's natural energy systems.

Equalizer Concentrate: Fulvic acid aids the body to dissolve toxins while enhancing nutritional absorption and cellular function. It is a powerful anti-viral, improves cellular communication and promotes immune system response.

Black Brew: Elements in this formula bond to heavy metals in the gut before they can be absorbed and enhance thyroid, liver, kidney and cardiovascular functions. Black Brew also helps with hormone balance and eye health.

INSTRUCTIONS FOR THE 3-DAY LIQUID DETOX

Make the vegetable broth early in the morning on day 1, or the previous day (overnight in a slow cooker works great). Use the Gut Healing Vegetable Broth recipe provided later in this book and be aware that you may have some broth left over. The broth and chamomile tea should help keep your belly satisfied.

We recommend that you make the juices fresh and drink them right away to get the highest nutritional and detoxifying effects. However, you can make the juices for the day, keep them in glass containers in the refrigerator, then drink them throughout the day.

If you do not have a juicer, you may be able to have these made at your health food store. Please make sure to ask if they use organic ingredients.

Never do a juicing detox with non-organic ingredients, especially with root vegetables! It will be counterproductive, or may give you large amounts of toxic chemicals, such as glyphosate. Glyphosate is a detrimental, toxic ingredient that is affecting everyone I know.

The following recipes can be found later in this book:

- Gut Healing Vegetable Broth
- Morning Melon Detox
- Deep in Red Detox
- Afternoon Orange Cleanser
- Fresh Pink Hydrator
- Evening Green Cleanse

Chamomile tea should be made from dried chamomile flowers. You can purchase bulk, dry chamomile flowers at your health food store or online. Make your tea with filtered water. You may add 1/2 teaspoon of honey per cup of tea, but be sure to limit your total honey to no more than 1 tablespoon per day.

THE DAILY ROUTINE (REPEAT EACH DAY):

Morning, 7-9 AM

- Start your day with 16 ounces of distilled or RO water.
- Take 1-2 Super Earth Energy, 4 sprays of Equalizer Concentrate, and 1/8 teaspoon of black brew mixed in distilled or RO water (optional).
- Make and drink Morning Melon Detox juice.
- One to two hours later: drink chamomile tea or veggie broth.

Midmorning (before noon)

- Make and drink Deep in Red Detox juice.
- One to two hours later: drink chamomile tea or veggie broth.

Afternoon, 1-2 p.m.

- Take 1-2 Super Earth Energy and 4 sprays of Equalizer Concentrate (optional).
- Make and drink Orange Afternoon Cleanse juice.
- One to two hours later: drink chamomile tea or veggie broth.

Early Afternoon

- Make and drink Fresh Pink Hydrator juice (use a blender to mix).
- One to two hours later: drink chamomile tea or veggie broth.

Evening (dinner time), 6-7 PM

- Take 1-2 Super Earth Energy, 4 sprays of Equalizer Concentrate, and 1/8 teaspoon of black brew mixed in distilled or RO water (optional).
- Make and drink Evening Green Cleanse juice.
- Feel free to drink chamomile tea before bed.

SHOPPING LIST FOR 3-DAY LIQUID DETOX

- Avocado oil
- 1 red onion
- 1 garlic bulb, large
- 1 cup kale
- 1 cup spinach
- Raw apple cider vinegar
- 7 bunches parsley
- Mixed veggies for veggie broth (carrots, cabbage, celery, mushrooms)
- 1/2 cup dried or fresh shiitake mushrooms
- 1 tablespoon whole peppercorns
- 2 tablespoons coconut aminos
- 1 bunch fresh coriander leaf (cilantro)
- 2 cantaloupes
- 1 watermelon
- 6 apples (at least 3 green)

- 1 large bunch grapes (3 cups total)
- 6 lemons
- 3 oranges
- 3 grapefruits (optional)
- 3 bunches celery (need 42 stalks for juices, plus more for veggie broth)
- 1 bunch of cherry tomatoes (optional)
- 3 red beets
- 5-6 bunches whole carrots (need at least 39 whole carrots for juices, plus more for veggie broth)
- 3 green onions
- 3 cucumbers
- Turmeric root (at least 3 inches), ground can be used for veggie broth
- Ginger root (7-8 inches total)

SELF-CARE WHILE ON A LIQUID FAST

While fasting on liquids, your body is in a compromised state. It may seem as though you should be feeling better than ever as your body is eliminating waste and toxicity from your system, but your body is actually working very hard to detoxify from the inside out. Take this time to rest and catch up on sleep, spend time in the sauna, go on a long walk, do meditation and deep breathing, soak in an Epsom salt bath, or practice gentle yoga moves or stretching exercises.

Pushing the body too hard while you are juicing may cause you to crash. It may allow for toxins to re-enter your system and result in fatigue and feeling sicker than before. I urge you to work gently with your body, particularly if you are struggling with detoxing.

OPTIONAL DURING THE 3-DAY LIQUID DETOX

Coffee enemas can be a great addition to your liquid fast. As an option, perform one coffee enema each day during your detox, early in the afternoon. This will help your entire system and take your detox to the next level. You can find instructions for doing a coffee enema later in the 21-Day Detox.

2-WEEK DETOX

This detox protocol is designed to break the cycle of irritation and inflammation by helping your body detoxify in a safe and beneficial way. It cleanses your liver, gallbladder, colon, intestines, and lymphatic system, making it a whole-body cleanse. Implementing this detox will reduce your body's need for cortisol (the stress hormone) by removing pro-inflammatory substances while at the same time enhancing insulin sensitivity.

WHO SHOULD DO THIS DETOX

This detox is great for anyone who wants to dedicate moderate time to do a deeper detox than the beginner and the 3-Day Liquid protocols. This is a perfect protocol to start after finishing the 3-Day protocol because your body will be primed to eliminate toxins. This is also perfect for someone who is dealing with stress, either externally or internally, or has dealt with high levels of stress throughout their lives.

FOODS TO EAT DURING THE 2-WEEK DETOX

During this program eat as many vegetables as you can—these foods are your main detoxifiers. You may also eat fruits, but limit them to no more than 1/3 cup of fruit for each full cup of vegetables you eat.

All of the recipes Gina created (in the last section of the book) are allowed while completing this protocol. You should not be hungry, as you will be eating plenty of food full of vital nutrients. You can also reference the "allowed foods" and "foods to avoid" from chapter seven if you wish to make your own detox dishes.

To maintain blood sugar levels, you will need to eat snacks between meals. I recommend fruits, vegetables, seaweed or kale chips, and nuts.

Suggested Fruits:

- Apples: at least 1 every day. You may eat more than 1, keeping in mind the fruit to vegetable ratio.
- Pears: 1 every other day.
- Berries: 1 cup every day or every other day.

SUPPLEMENTS

Incorporating supplements in this detox protocol is an option; however, the effectiveness of the detox is maximized when including them. Listed below are supplements specific to this 2-Week Detox and all can be found at DrNuzum.com.

Equalizer Concentrate: Fulvic Acid aids the body in dissolving toxins while enhancing nutritional absorption and cellular function. It is a powerful antiviral, improves cellular communication, and promotes healthy immune system response.

Black Brew: Elements in this formula bond to heavy metals in the gut before they can be absorbed and enhance thyroid, liver, kidney, and cardiovascular functions. Black Brew also helps with hormone balance and eye health.

Super Curcuminoids: This formula helps regulate inflammatory enzymes, promotes a healthy immune system, maintains a healthy digestive tract, and supports every organ system.

Digestive Detox: This formula contains potent seeds and herbs to cleanse your whole digestive tract and a pre-biotic, pro-biotic blend to combat the unhealthy bacteria in the colon. This combination supports the health of the intestinal membranes while building a healthy immune system.

Aloe vera juice, cold-pressed: Found at the local health food store. Ensure it has no added ingredients. Aloe vera is an anti-inflammatory and aids in digestion and healing leaky gut and intestinal membranes. It also helps with lowering cholesterol and lubricates the intestinal tract, which facilitates detoxification and acts as a prebiotic.

THE DAILY ROUTINE

Morning

- Upon waking, drink 8 ounces of pure water with 1/8 teaspoon Black Brew.
- Take 4 sprays of Equalizer Concentrate. You may spray Equalizer Concentrate straight into your mouth, or add it to juice, tea, or water.
- Before breakfast, make and drink a Cleansing Cocktail (recipe on next page).
- Drink 1 ounce cold-pressed aloe vera juice.

Noon

- Before your midday meal, make and drink Cleansing Cocktail and take 4 sprays of Equalizer Concentrate.
- Take 4 Super Curcuminoids with your meal.

Evening

- Try to avoid eating dinner after 7 p.m.
- Make and drink Cleansing Cocktail before dinner and take 4 sprays of Equalizer Concentrate.

Before Bed

- Take 1/8 teaspoon of Black Brew powder, 4 ounces of pure water, and 4 capsules of Digestive Detox.

- If you're feeling hungry, try drinking a cup of chamomile tea. You can also eat a kiwi with a handful of almonds or half of an apple with nut butter.

ESSENTIAL SHOPPING LIST

Your full shopping list will vary depending on what recipes you decide to make, but here is a list for one week of items that are essential to starting the detox program.

- Raw, organic apple cider vinegar (such as Bragg's)
- Organic honey, raw or unfiltered
- 3-5 organic lemons
- 4 organic pears
- Organic berries for the whole 2 weeks
- 7 organic apples
- Filtered or RO water

CLEANSING COCKTAIL RECIPE

- 1 teaspoon fresh lemon juice
- 1 teaspoon organic raw apple cider vinegar
- 1 teaspoon honey (raw or unfiltered)
- 1 cup distilled or reverse osmosis water

If this is not palatable you may add 3/4 cup of organic apple juice. You may drink it cold also, if preferred.

NOTES

Relax. Stress causes the adrenal glands to produce a hormone called cortisol. A little cortisol is necessary to initiate the detox process in your body, but too much slows down the process and causes you to crave sugar, gain weight, retain water, and feel fatigued. Stress is one of the most toxic and deteriorating factors that we face. Decreasing stress will enhance your body's ability to detoxify. Consider meditation, a daily walk, light exercise, a bath, a nap, or quiet time to give back to your body and decrease stress. Whatever you choose to do to de-stress will reduce your cortisol levels.

Coffee is not allowed during this program because it raises cortisol levels, stresses the adrenal glands, and will contribute to sugar cravings. Weaning off coffee can cause you to be somewhat lethargic and tired, which is typical for about three days. You may experience headaches, but drinking green and other herbal teas throughout the day can help alleviate the cravings and withdrawals. Rooibos tea is an excellent replacement for coffee.

21-DAY DETOX

The 21-Day Detox is similar to the 2-Week Detox protocol, but adds time, extra supplementation and cleansing activities to increase your overall toxin elimination. This hard core detox protocol takes a bit more mental fortitude as well.

WHO SHOULD DO THIS DETOX

The 21-Day Detox is for the more seasoned veterans of the detoxification world. It is the toughest detox program that I use, but is also the most effective. Detoxing for 21 days gives you additional benefits such as weight loss, metabolic rehabilitation, and behavioral modification.

Anyone who has time to dedicate to a serious detox and may need thorough cleansing of all systems will want to do this protocol. I recommend completing a 2-Week Detox protocol prior to starting in order to more fully prepare for this more intense version.

FOODS TO EAT DURING THE 21-DAY DETOX

Follow the same diet plan from my 2-Week Detox. Basically, any of the foods included in the recipes section of this book are allowed. They will provide an abundant variety of flavors and should help keep your taste buds satisfied. You can also reference the "allowed foods" and "foods to avoid" from chapter seven if you wish to make your own detox dishes. Finally, maintain the veggie to fruit to protein ratio of 60-20-20.

SUPPLEMENTS

Super Earth Energy: This formula supports the adrenal and thyroid glands as well as the body's natural energy systems.

Digestive Detox: This formula contains potent seeds and herbs to cleanse your whole digestive tract and a pre-biotic, pro-biotic blend to combat the unhealthy bacteria in the colon. This combination supports the health of the intestinal membranes while building a healthy immune system.

Black Brew: Elements in this formula bond to heavy metals in the gut before they can be absorbed and enhance thyroid, liver, kidney, and cardiovascular functions. Black Brew also helps with hormone balance and eye health.

Inflamagone: A combination of the most powerful anti-inflammatory botanical medicines to reduce inflammation, enhance circulatory function, support microbial balance, protect DNA, and aid in the rebuilding of joints and bones.

Super Chlorogenic: This chlorogenic acid formula is a natural antioxidant and liver supporter that aids in weight loss, promotes metabolic health, helps the cardiovascular system, and helps the liver to release stored sugar.

THE DAILY ROUTINE

Days 1-10

Morning

- Take Super Earth Energy: 3 capsules
- Take Inflamagone: 2 capsules
- Take Super Chlorogenic: 1 capsule
- Take Black Brew: 1/8 teaspoon mixed in distilled or RO water

Noon

- Take Super Earth Energy: 2 capsules
- Take Inflamagone: 3 capsules
- Take Super Chlorogenic: 1 capsule

Afternoon

- Take Super Chlorogenic: 1 capsule
- Take Digestive Detox: 3 capsules
- Take Black Brew: 1/8 teaspoon mixed in distilled or RO water
- (No Super Earth Energy or Inflamagone)

Day 11

Discontinue all supplements for this one day only.

Also, you must fast this day. No food.

You may drink distilled or RO water, but make sure you also consume the following throughout the day:

Throughout day but before 8 PM, consume:

- 48 oz. of organic chamomile tea, with a small amount of organic honey and the fresh juice of 1 lemon per 24 oz. of tea
- 48 oz. of organic apple juice

After 8 PM, prepare the following:

- Mix 3 oz. of organic extra-virgin olive oil and 3 oz. of fresh-squeezed organic lemon juice
- Drink all of the mixture, then lay on your **right** side for 30 minutes

Drinking these specific mixtures signals the gallbladder to expel its contents, which is the primary benefit. This often includes expelling gallstones.

Days 12-21

Continue eating food from recipes in the back of this book, or follow the "allowed foods" list in chapter seven.

Continue taking supplements as follows:

Morning

- Take Super Earth Energy: 3 capsules
- Take Inflamagone: 2 capsules
- Take Super Chlorogenic: 1 capsule
- Take Black Brew: 1/8 teaspoon mixed in distilled or RO water

Noon

- Take Super Earth Energy: 2 capsules
- Take Inflamagone: 3 capsules
- Take Super Chlorogenic: 1 capsule

Afternoon

- Take Super Chlorogenic: 1 capsule
- Take Digestive Detox: 3 capsules
- Take Black Brew: 1/8 teaspoon mixed in distilled or RO water
- (No Super Earth Energy or Inflamagone)

ADDITIONAL ACTIVITIES

Detox Baths

Every other day for the entire 21 days, take a detox bath:

- 2 cups Epsom salt
- 2 cups Baking Soda
- 2 cups hydrogen peroxide

Mix above ingredients into water as tub is filling. Soak in hot bath for 30 minutes.

Coffee Enemas

It is extremely important to use quality organic coffee for your coffee enema to avoid harmful chemicals such as pesticides and herbicides. Because of the high demand of regular coffee, it is grown in a very toxic and polluted manner.

This procedure includes **2 enemas**: a warm water enema followed by a coffee enema.

You will need:

- Reusable enema kit
- 16 ounces of warm distilled water
- 16 ounces of warm organic, fair-trade brewed coffee (preferably dark coffee bean)

Every third day for the entire 21 days, perform this coffee enema:

Brew the coffee:

- Brew 16 ounces of organic coffee with distilled water. These are the only two ingredients that should be used.
- Allow to cool to lukewarm. Do not ever take a hot coffee enema. You can burn your colon, which is very dangerous and can be very harmful to your lower intestinal health.

Administer the distilled water enema first, followed by the warm, organic coffee.

For the enemas:

- Pour lukewarm distilled water or coffee into an enema bag. Hang the enema bag at the same level of your head.
- Kneel on all fours and insert the nozzle of the enema tube into your anus. Keep pressure on the tube so that the coffee cannot escape the enema bag.
- Allow the coffee to flow freely into rectum and retain for as long as possible, then evacuate. The longer you retain the coffee, the deeper the cleansing action.

Coffee is an excellent substance for detoxifying the liver. Coffee enemas will stimulate the dilation of the common bile duct, as well as the sphincter. This helps the liver to drain itself more effectively. You may expel large quantities of "stones" when doing a coffee enema. Coffee enemas are contraindicated, or questionable, for those with ulcerative colitis, bleeding hemorrhoids (both internal and external), and Crohn's disease. Most people can do coffee enemas and benefit from them greatly. After finishing the 21-Day Detox, it is important that you only administer an enema two times a month or not more than one time weekly.

Tips for successful coffee enemas:

- Do not use light roast coffee for enemas—they are too thin.
- Do not use cold liquid as it can cause severe cramping.
- Start with only an ounce of coffee, just in case you are sensitive to it.
- Cleanliness is extremely important when involving the pelvis. Wash everything carefully with soap and water after use.

- Before applying the enema, make sure the coffee is not hot which will burn and damage the membranes in the colon, and not too cold which will cause cramping.

- Never force the enema tip into the rectum. Lubricate it well with coconut oil or olive oil and move it slowly and gently, aiming it directly upward. Be sure it goes all the way in.

- Never retain the enema if the pressure to release it is too high. Listen to your body.

- Act with care, don't force anything.

- The experience of an enema can be unnerving. It takes practice to get accustomed to it.

- Start with smaller quantities of coffee and increase with each enema until you reach the 16 ounce range.

- Distilled water is best for coffee enemas. If this is not available, you can use reverse osmosis, or at least carbon-only filtered tap water.

- French press or boiling water poured over the ground coffee is the best way to brew the coffee. This way you avoid contaminants and chemicals.

END OF 21-DAY PROTOCOL

If you are completing one of our detox protocols and have questions, please email us at detox@drnuzum.com.

Also, if you want support from others who are detoxing, or from people who have previously completed one of our detox protocols, join our Facebook group, *Detox Your Way to Health.*

AFTER A DETOX PROTOCOL

Congratulations—you did it!

You just gave your body a great gift by ridding it of harmful toxins. For the next few days, slowly reintroduce foods back into your diet and continue to drink plenty of water. Pay close attention to any foods that may cause a reaction such as runny nose, headache or stomachache, pain, mood change, or needing to go to the bathroom immediately. If dairy, gluten, grains, or meat causes any of these reactions, it may be time to remove them from your diet.

> "Let thy food be thy medicine and thy medicine be thy food."
> —Hippocrates, the father of medicine

I highly recommend that you stay on a healthy diet, eating mostly from the "allowed foods" list. Besides detoxifying your body, we hope that going through one of these programs helped tune you in to your body's signals and discover some changes that need to be made to your diet. For some people, it may have been simple to eat mostly vegetables, but it's understandable that for others it was a big change, and very difficult. Changing your diet for the better can take some time and you will need to give yourself plenty of grace.

Maya Angelou said, "Do the best you can until you know better. Then when you know better, do better." This is a wonderful quote to remember as you make your next health decisions.

Depending on your state of health, these detox programs can be done every season, every three months, or every other month as a way to reboot your filters. Check with your natural healthcare provider to help you develop a plan.

You may have some supplements left over after the detox is finished. Feel free to take them until they're gone. The Equalizer Concentrate is one product you should not be without, as it is an ongoing cellular regenerator and detoxifier. If you want additional supplements for daily maintenance, visit DrNuzum.com and consider the following:

- Super Earth Energy
- Equalizer Concentrate

You can also find more programs and protocols for issues like inflammation and energy at DrNuzum.com under the "Protocols" tab.

Every day you have the choice to build and nourish your body—make it a good choice!

DETOX AS A LIFESTYLE

As I've said several times throughout this book, some of the toxins you encounter in your life cannot be avoided. But you can choose to avoid many, many kinds of toxins and in doing that, support your body and its ability to protect you from those things you can't control.

Eating nutritious, organic foods and drinking pure water is better for you and the environment. Plus, you positively impact the lives of organic farmers and retailers by choosing to eat organic, non-GMO foods. This all helps you remain positive because you are giving your body what it needs to adapt to those uncontrollable conditions—restoring a little power back to you.

When you understand that food truly is medicine, you can easily turn away from junk food and choose to eat what nourishes you and the planet. You can continue to move your body in the direction of health. The demand for organic food is growing, and every acre, every farm that converts to organic practices is one more that isn't contributing to environmental contamination. Doing this while you support your body to live in health is a win for everyone.

Detox as a lifestyle means minimizing your exposure to toxins and maximizing your ability to deal with what you can't avoid.

Detox for life means educating yourself, and staying educated about air, water, and food conditions, as well as choosing to support organizations that support health and life. This book is filled with knowledge about how to stabilize your body and environment, how to recognize how toxins are disrupting your body, and how to detoxify and fortify your body for optimal health.

In the final section, I will yield to my wife Gina to further educate you on some very delicious ways to continue to fortify your body with food. All of her recipes are healthy, nutrient rich, and life-giving dishes that can be enjoyed during a detox or any time. She provides creative, delicious recipes to inspire your own creativity in eating for your life and your health. Turn the page for beautiful and nutritious eating.

Patient Story

2-Week Detox Testimonial

I went through Dr. Nuzum's 2-Week Detox program more than once and ultimately, it changes everything for the better. My skin clears up. My hair and nails become stronger and shinier. My eyesight improves and the straining headaches I get from looking at computer screens for long hours subside. I sleep better. My respiratory system clears up. I used to get ear infections and nasal infections pretty regularly and anytime that comes on, I will do another regimen and it clears up. I find that my drive for life increases from doing this kind of thing intermittently and I have more patience and endurance for stressors in my life. I have been able to move my metabolic set point to where it is easier to maintain a healthier weight that is about fifteen to twenty pounds less than before I started taking Dr Nuzum's advice. I also sleep a lot better and interestingly enough, I have been able to remember my dreams more clearly.

I also use several of Dr. Nuzum's supplements, but I would like to call attention to my favorites. His Super Earth Energy supplement is one that I have used non-stop ever since I first tried it. This mineral supplement is beyond compare and I remember when he took the time to go down the list of all the ingredients and their qualities, as well as the synergy with my second favorite, his fulvic acid.

Fulvic acid is used in many of his products because unlike any other supplements, that one delivers the nutrients through the cell walls. I use Equalizer Concentrate sublingually in concert with other supplements. Finally, the black brew is a humic acid supplement that I now use every day in the morning in my yerba mate tea. This cleansing supplement draws heavy metals, radiation, and toxins out and along with his cleansing programs, this one really seals the deal, making the detoxification experience far more effective than anything else.

—Chad G.

See some of the recipes Chad submitted, starting on page 236.

PART 3: FORTIFY

Detox Diet Recipes

DETOX DIET RECIPES

Hi, Gina here, welcome to the fun part of this book—the recipe section!

I am a busy mom of 5 who loves to cook and create healthy recipes. Being married to my amazing husband has taught me a lot about natural medicine, and using nature to support the body to find harmony. After many pregnancies, exposure to toxins and heavy metals, and working through the loss of our baby, I fell into thyroid crisis from so many stressful situations. Dan helped me understand how the body works and how food is medicine. He had me complete the 2-Week Detox, put me on a supplement regimen, and I only ate healthy foods as "prescribed."

Thankfully, I feel so much better now and continue to see improvements every day. My health crisis has allowed me to have even more compassion for all of the patients that seek our help, as I know what they are going through. It is important to find support and encouragement when we don't feel well. It's also very helpful to find a "tribe" when making significant changes to your lifestyle.

The first time I did the 2-Week Detox protocol, I felt like a rabbit! I didn't have a good variety of food to keep me satisfied, so I decided to create recipes that would be "allowed" while doing a detox. I didn't want anyone else to struggle through a protocol because their taste buds were bored. Plus, I knew if I made delicious recipes, people would want to incorporate them into their regular meal plans, not just while on a detox. This is really the ultimate goal, to shift to detoxifying and fortifying, nutritious foods as a lifestyle.

While I was detoxing, several patients from our clinic were detoxing too, so we were constantly texting and chatting about our experience. As we started sharing recipes, I realized it would be great support to start a Facebook group so all of our patients could be part of a detox tribe. So, I started Detox Your Way to Health to stay in touch with those going through our detox programs. Please join in the discussions, whether you are currently detoxing or not, everyone always learns from the group and I hope it provides support to everyone who participates.

I hope you find support through this book as well. I was lucky to have a mom who spent hours in the kitchen teaching me how to cook. I know it may not be like having the support of a mom, but take this book in the kitchen to accompany you through your healthy cooking journey. Relax, put on some music, and get creative! Find some recipes you love, keep making them, then create some of your own. Share them with your friends and for sure, share them in the Detox Your Way to Health Facebook group using the hashtag #nuzumsdetox.

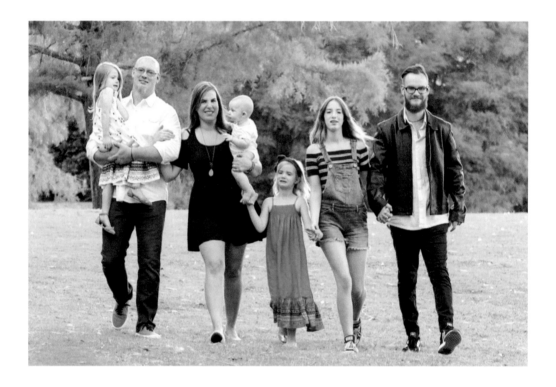

From our family to yours—Doc and I wish you the best of
health and vitality for life!

Juices

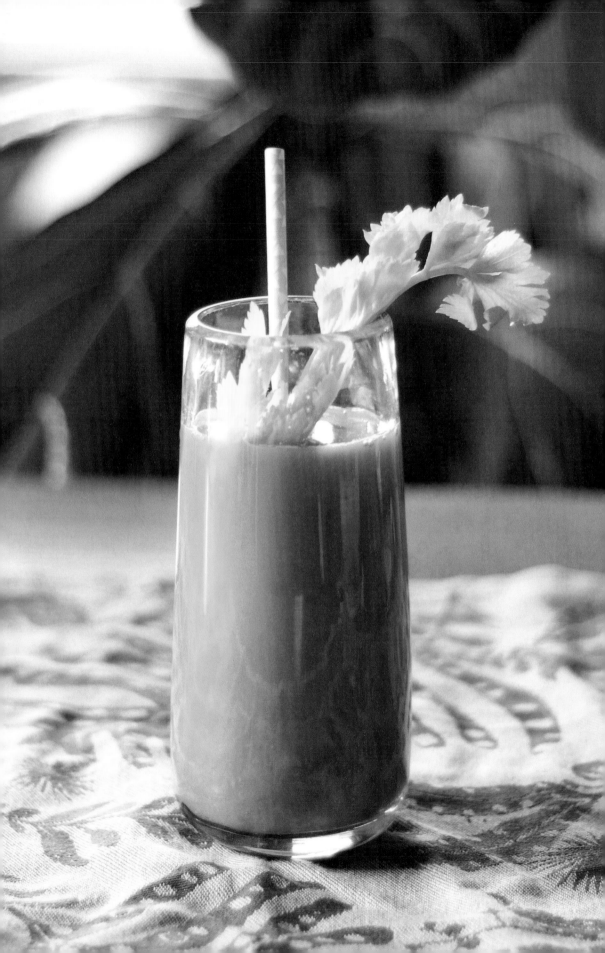

Morning Melon Detox

INGREDIENTS:

1/2 small cantaloupe without seeds

1 apple

3 celery stalks

3 carrots

1/2 ounce ginger root

1/2 ounce turmeric root

1 cucumber

DIRECTIONS:

Process all ingredients through a quality juicer. Prep time and clean-up time are both approximately 10 minutes.

• • • • •

Juicing gives the body a break from digesting heavy foods and helps cleanse it in a gentle way. This section kicks off some of our favorite juices that are approved for our 3-Day Liquid Detox program.

BENEFITS OF GINGER:

A powerful anti-inflammatory, antioxidant, and overall healing root, ginger is also an excellent detoxifier. Ginger expels phlegm and toxic waste from the lungs, enhances liver detoxification, detoxifies the kidneys, and stimulates all aspects of digestion.

Total Time: 15-20 min.
Serves: 1-2

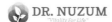

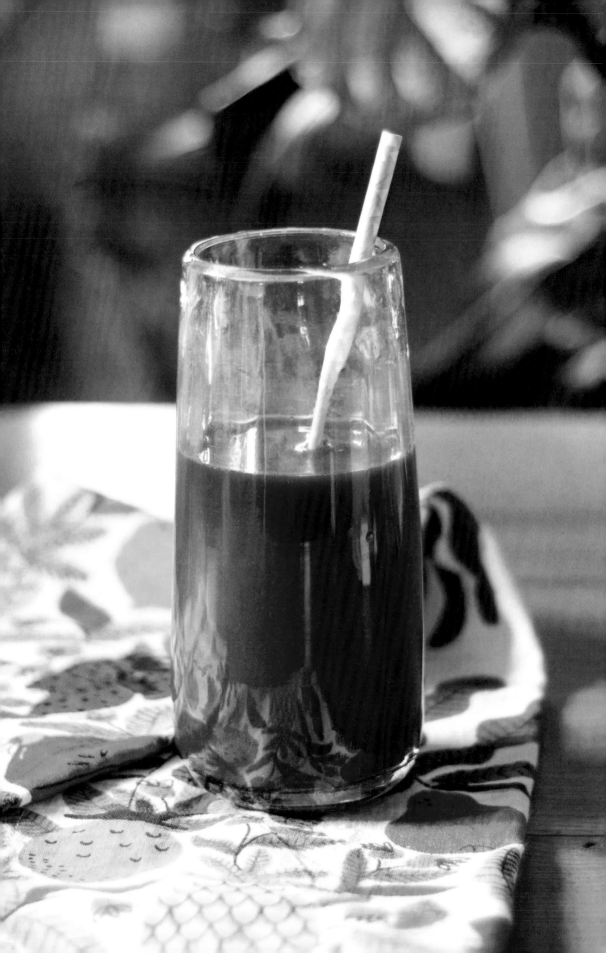

Deep in Red Detox

INGREDIENTS:

1/2 to 1 red beet

4 medium carrots

4 celery stalks

1 apple

1/2 to 1 inch ginger root

OPTIONS:

Juice of one grapefruit

DIRECTIONS:

Process all ingredients through a quality juicer. Prep time and clean-up time are both approximately 10 minutes.

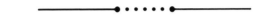

Juicing can help reduce inflammation in the body, especially this recipe with its highly anti-inflammatory beets.

BENEFITS OF BEETS:

Various acids and nutrients in beets cleanse bile ducts in the liver, allowing waste to leave the liver more efficiently. Beets are excellent for liver cleansing and improving circulation, while acting as a natural anti-inflammatory.

Total Time: 15-20 min.
Serves: 1

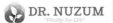

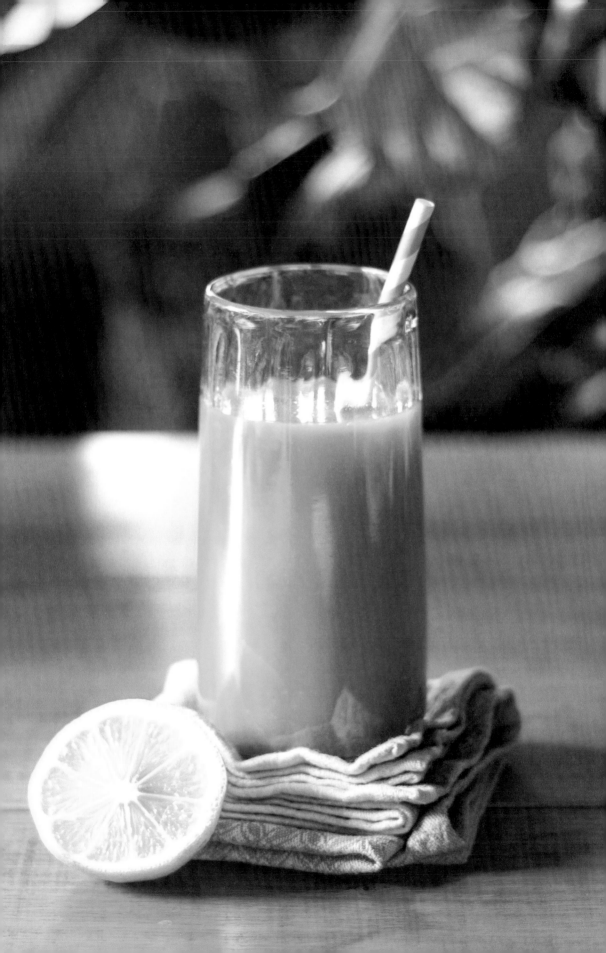

Afternoon Orange Cleanser

INGREDIENTS:

1 lemon with some peel

1 orange with some peel

3 carrots

1/2 inch piece of ginger root

1/2 inch piece of fresh turmeric root

1 green onion

DIRECTIONS:

Process all ingredients through a quality juicer. Prep time and clean-up time are both approximately 10 minutes.

Note: Turmeric root is usually found in the same area of the grocery store where fresh ginger is found. While it's great to use fresh turmeric, sometimes it's hard to find. If you don't have fresh turmeric, you can substitute turmeric powder. Add the powder after the ingredients have been processed through the juicer. The flavor will be slightly different, but it's better than leaving it out altogether.

———— ● · · · · ● ————

Never do a juicing detox with non-organic roots such as the carrots, ginger, and turmeric in this recipe, as it will be counterproductive to detoxification. Always use organic!

BENEFITS OF TURMERIC:

Turmeric is a liver protector and an ancient anti-inflammatory root that belongs to the ginger family. It contains phytochemicals called curcuminoids that provide a wide array of health benefits. Most notably, curcuminoids support brain and cardiovascular health as well as help relieve pain and stiffness in joints.

Total Time: 15-20 min.
Serves: 1

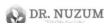

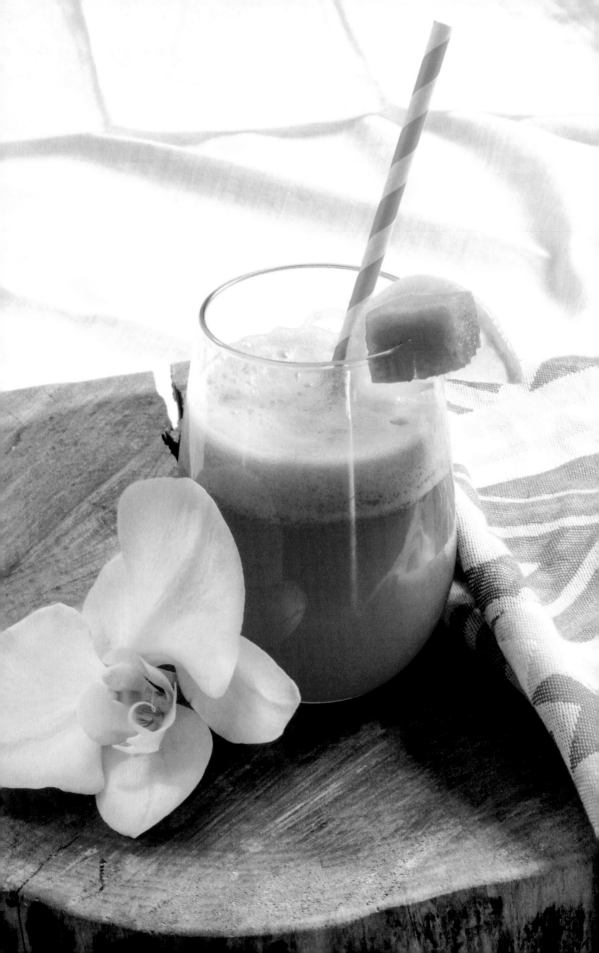

Fresh Pink Hydrator

INGREDIENTS:

1/4 large or 1/2 small watermelon

Juice of one lemon

1 cup water (may add more water if desired)

DIRECTIONS:

Blend all ingredients in high-speed blender until smooth.

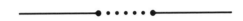

This juice is one of the simplest to make and is also one of the most familiar for the taste buds, especially for those doing a juice cleanse for the first time.

BENEFITS OF WATERMELON:

The high water content in watermelon—92 percent—makes it an incredibly hydrating thirst quencher. Watermelon is also high in calcium and potassium, which helps lower the risk of high blood pressure. Watermelon contains vitamin A, which is good for eye health, contains immune system supporting vitamin C, and has a cleansing effect on the kidneys. When it comes to cancer prevention and treatment, the lycopene in watermelon has been shown to interrupt the growth of cancer cells.

Total Time: 5 min.
Serves: 1-2

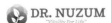

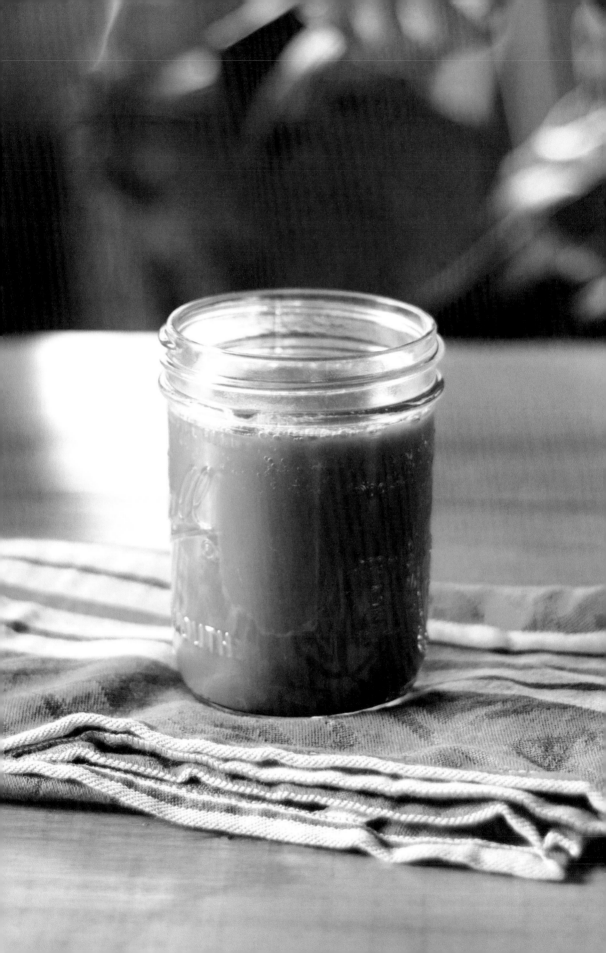

Evening Green Cleanse

INGREDIENTS:

6-7 celery stalks

3 carrots

1/2 ounce ginger root

1 green apple

1 large bunch parsley

1 cup grapes

DIRECTIONS:

Process all ingredients through a quality juicer. Prep time and clean-up time are both approximately 10 minutes.

• • • • •

Naturally occurring live enzymes that are derived from raw juices add to your enzyme bank, making juicing a beneficial detoxing asset. Any foods cooked over 116° destroy the naturally occurring enzymes. When we eat cooked foods, our bodies are forced to use large amounts of stored enzymes, depleting the body of these precious chemical catalysts.

BENEFITS OF GRAPES:

The polyphenols found in grapes are powerful antioxidants that can aid in cancer prevention. According to Chinese Medicine, grapes nourish the blood and strengthen bones and tendons. They also have an expectorant effect, which means they help thin mucus in the lungs. Strong antioxidant and anti-inflammatory qualities in grapes support the cardiovascular system, and the low glycemic index value helps with blood sugar balance and insulin regulation.

Total Time: 15-20 min.
Serves: 1

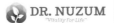

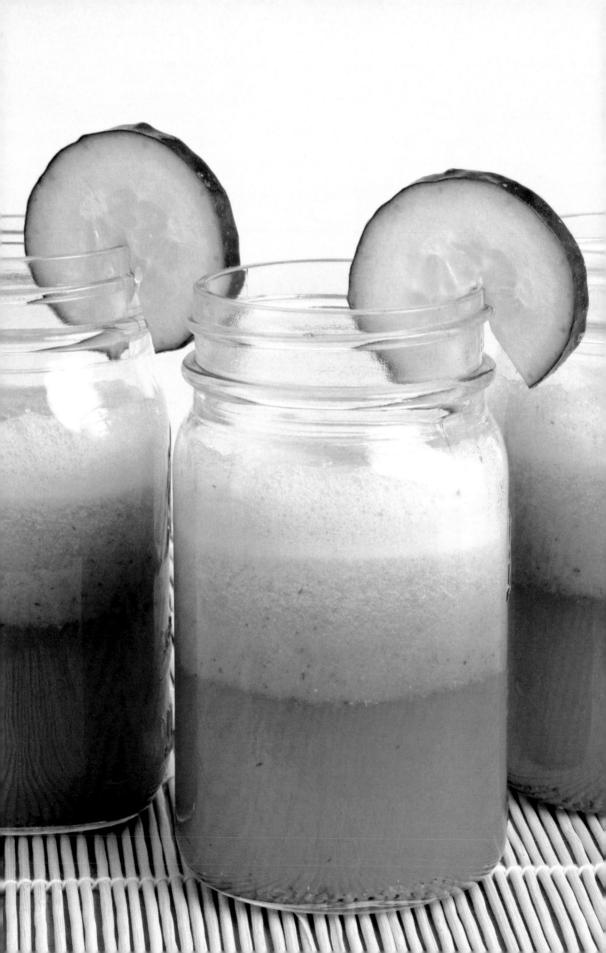

Cucumber Refresher

INGREDIENTS:

1 large lemon juiced, with some peel

1/2 large cucumber, washed with peel

1 tablespoon honey

5 cups water

Cucumber slices for garnish

DIRECTIONS:

Blend all ingredients in a high-speed blender for about one minute.

———————— ● • • • • ● ————————

This drink can be served over ice, or made into ice cubes to be served with water. If you choose to make ice cubes, double the recipe.

BENEFITS OF CUCUMBER:

Belonging to the same plant family as watermelon, cucumber is sure to keep you cool on a hot day. Cucumbers contain important electrolytes, magnesium, and potassium, and its 95 percent water content is important for deep hydration. The peel and seeds contain beta carotene, fiber, and calcium, which boosts immunity and promotes healthy eyes, skin, hair, and nails.

Total Time: 5 min.
Serves: 2-3

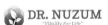
DR. NUZUM
"Vitality For Life"

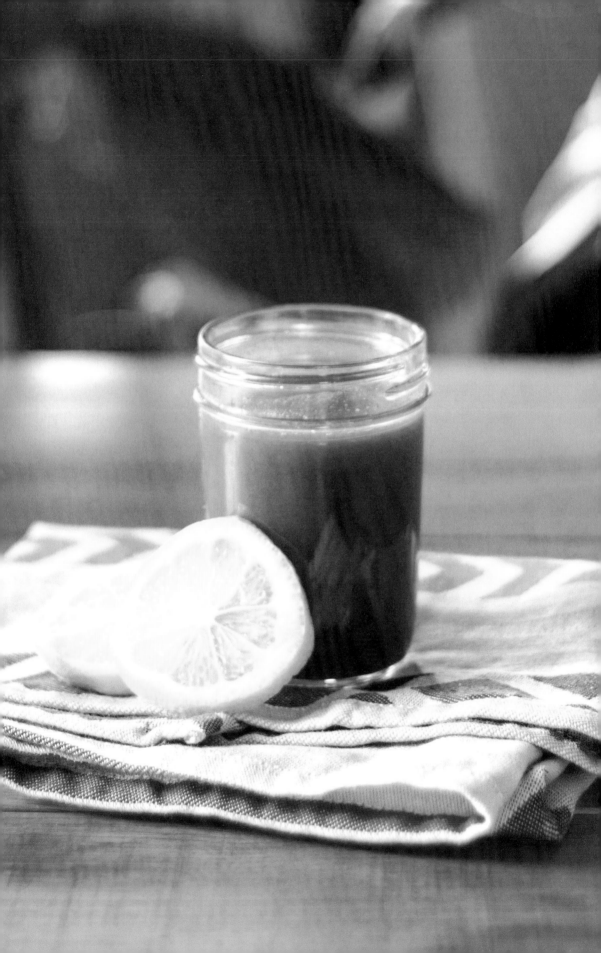

Wheatgrass Lemonade Energizer

INGREDIENTS:

2 lemons, juiced

2 teaspoons organic wheatgrass powder

1 tablespoon honey

5 cups water

DIRECTIONS:

Blend well and serve cold.

• • • • • •

The Energizer can be served over ice on a hot summer day. This is what Doc Nuzum drinks when he cuts the grass in the summer, and now, even our 16 year old son Daniel drinks this!

BENEFITS OF WHEATGRASS:

This juice is refreshing and full of nutrients, chlorophyll, vitamins, and minerals. Wheatgrass can help the body detoxify and should be consumed on an empty stomach or with fruits and vegetables. If consumed with a heavy meal, you may not feel well afterward. Wheatgrass can be used as a daily detoxifier.

Total Time: 5 min.
Serves: 2-3

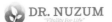

Smoothies

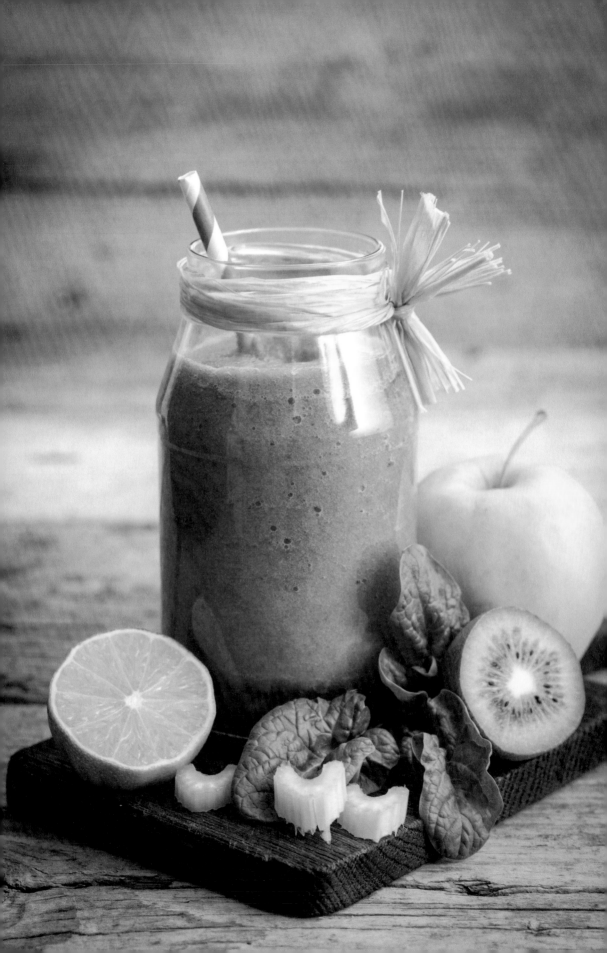

Green Apple

INGREDIENTS:

1 green apple

1 kiwi, peeled

1/2 cucumber

1 cup spinach

1 celery stalk, cut into pieces

1 1/2 cup filtered water

1/2 lime, juiced

1 cup ice

1 banana

OPTIONS:

1 collard green leaf for extra nutrients

Replace 1/2 cup water with organic green tea for added antioxidants and extra energy

1 tablespoon soaked chia seeds

DIRECTIONS:

Add all ingredients to a high-speed blender and blend until smooth.

Depending on your type of blender and desired thickness, you may need to add some extra water.

———— • • • • • ————

This is definitely a beginner's green smoothie that even children will enjoy. Sometimes it's hard for children, or even adults, to want to eat or drink something green, but when you show them the green apple and tell them it's a smoothie, it helps make the concept acceptable—certainly more acceptable than a parsley or spinach smoothie!

BENEFITS OF KIWI:

Packing more vitamin C than an orange, the kiwifruit is a nutritional powerhouse. The skin of the kiwi—yes, you can eat the skin if the fruit is organic— is also nutrient rich. The kiwi is high in omega–3 fatty acids which promotes mobility in joints and tendons. The kiwi is also rich in vitamins A, B6, B12, C, E, K, copper and potassium, rich in heart-healthy polyphenols, supports the health of the brain and immune system, and protects against free radical damage.

Total Time: 5 min.
Serves: 2-4

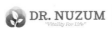

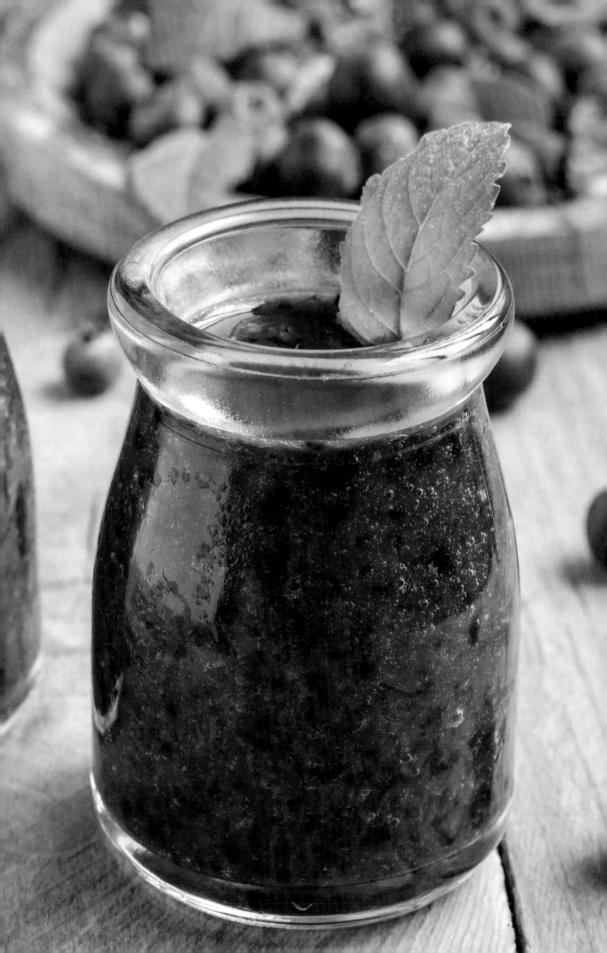

Blueberry Blast

INGREDIENTS:

1 cup frozen blueberries

Handful of fresh basil leaves

1 cup hemp or almond milk

3 ice cubes

1 teaspoon honey or pure maple syrup

OPTIONS:

Chia seeds

Unsweetened coconut flakes

DIRECTIONS:

Add all ingredients to a high speed blender and blend until smooth.

Depending on your type of blender and desired thickness, you may need to add some extra water.

Top with chia seeds, coconut flakes, or fresh mint if desired.

———————•••••••———————

This smoothie is very refreshing and surprisingly filling. It would be a great breakfast paired with a handful of almonds, or a perfect snack by itself.

BENEFITS OF BLUEBERRIES:

Blueberries are rich in vitamins such as calcium, magnesium, manganese, antioxidants, zinc, and vitamin K. They support digestion, improve insulin and glucose levels, improve cardiovascular health, and give the brain a boost.

> Total Time: 5 min.
> Serves: 2-4

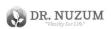

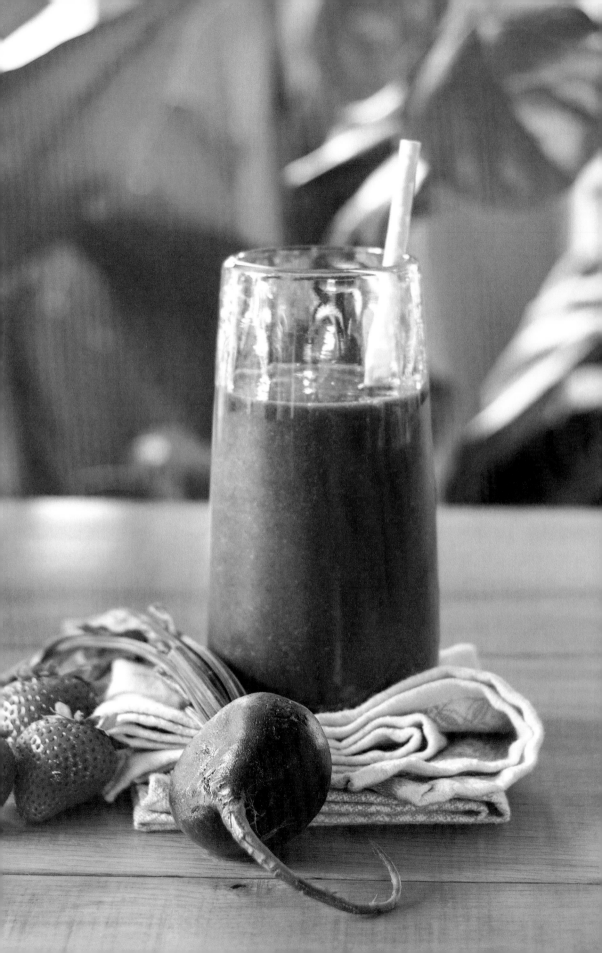

Strawberry Beet

INGREDIENTS:

1 cup frozen strawberries

1/4 cup frozen cherries

1/2 peeled banana

1/4 inch thick slice raw beet

1 cup Ice

1/2 cup water

OPTIONS:

1 teaspoon honey or stevia for extra sweetness

If you don't have frozen cherries, add extra strawberries

DIRECTIONS:

Add all ingredients to a high speed blender and blend until smooth.

Depending on your type of blender and desired thickness, you may need to add extra water.

· · · · ·

This is a delicious, vibrant, glowing smoothie—almost fluorescent from the beet pigment. And believe it or not, it does not taste "beety" at all. I dare you to try it! If you dislike beets, you can use a thinner slice and forget that it's in there.

If someone in your family doesn't like beets, make this smoothie and don't tell them the ingredients. Their liver will thank you!

BENEFITS OF BANANAS:

Bananas are probably most well known for being a good source of potassium. Potassium is an important mineral our body needs to maintain fluid levels and to regulate movement of nutrients and waste products in and out of cells. Additionally, potassium can help control the impact of sodium on blood pressure and may reduce the risk of forming kidney stones.

Total Time: 5 min.
Serves: 1

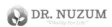

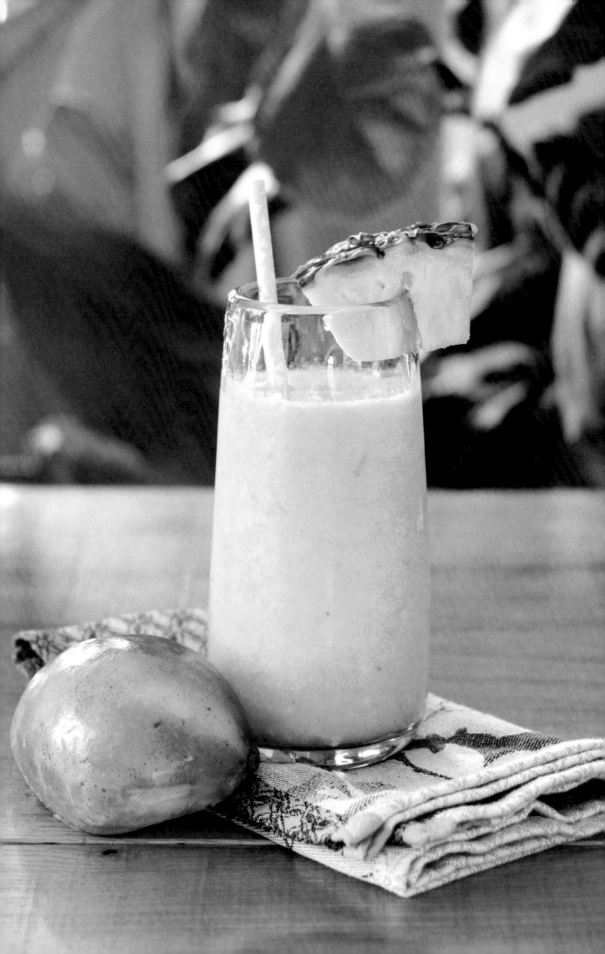

Tropical Sunshine

INGREDIENTS:

1/2 cup pineapple, cubed

1/2 banana, peeled

1/2 cup mango, peeled and cubed

1 cup ice

1/2 cup water

OPTIONS:

1/2 cup water to thin

1 teaspoon honey or stevia for extra sweetness

DIRECTIONS:

Cut skin off of pineapple and cut around the core to get fruit.

Add all ingredients to a high speed blender and blend until smooth.

Depending on your type of blender and desired thickness, you may need to add some extra water.

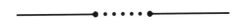

Smoothies are a great way to add many fruits and vegetables to your diet in one sitting—they are handy to take on-the-go.

BENEFITS OF MANGOES:

Mangoes are an excellent source of antioxidants and contribute to healthy eyes, skin, and mucous membranes. Mangoes have been shown to help prevent or halt the development of certain breast cancer and colon cancer cell lines—sending them into apoptosis (cell death) in lab studies. According to Chinese Medicine, mangoes can soothe a cough, regenerate fluids in the body, and strengthen digestion. The vitamin E assists in hormone regulation, the iron content contributes to healthy blood, and the mineral content of mangoes helps strengthen the bones.

Total Time: 5 min.
Serves: 3

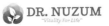

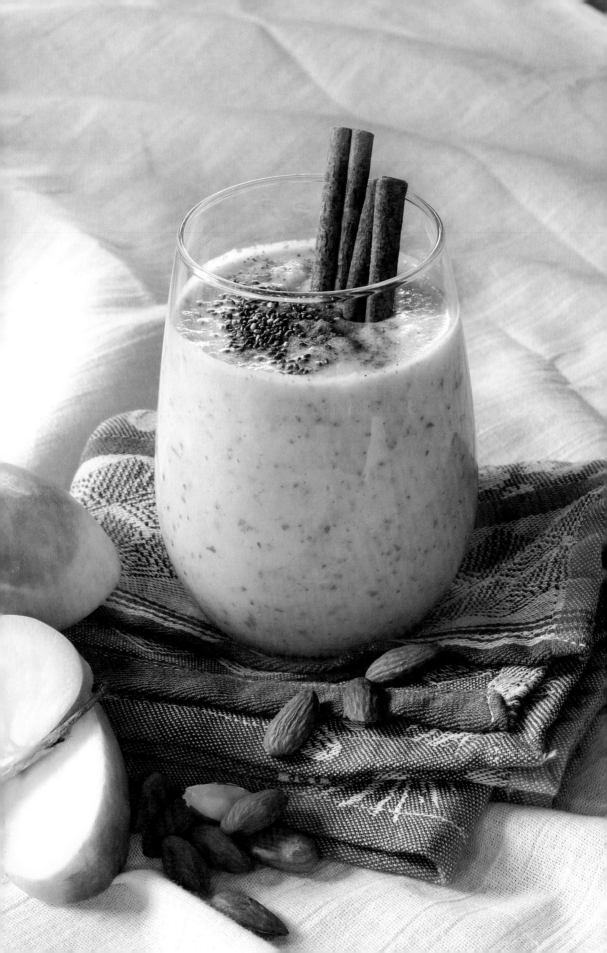

Apple Almond Glory

INGREDIENTS:

1 apple

1/4 cup almonds

1 cup hemp milk

1/2 cup water

1/4 teaspoon cinnamon

1/4 teaspoon vanilla extract

Pinch of Himalayan pink salt

4 ice cubes

OPTIONS:

Bee pollen

Chia seeds

It's best to soak the almonds for 12 hours, but you can add them without soaking if you don't have time.

DIRECTIONS:

Add all ingredients to a high-speed blender and blend until smooth.

Depending on your type of blender and desired thickness, you may need to add extra water.

Top with bee pollen or chia seeds if desired.

— • • • • • —

This is a delicious smoothie that my entire family loves. Sometimes I add a banana to it for a slight change in thickness and flavor. I always keep these ingredients at home so we can always whip up an apple almond glory. We hope you enjoy it as much as we do!

BENEFITS OF APPLES:

Apples are rich in antioxidants, high in fiber, and are anti-inflammatory. They help lower cholesterol, improve brain health, reduce the risk of colon, lung, and prostate cancer, and help prevent Alzheimer's disease.

Total Time: 5 min.
Serves: 1

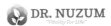

Breakfast

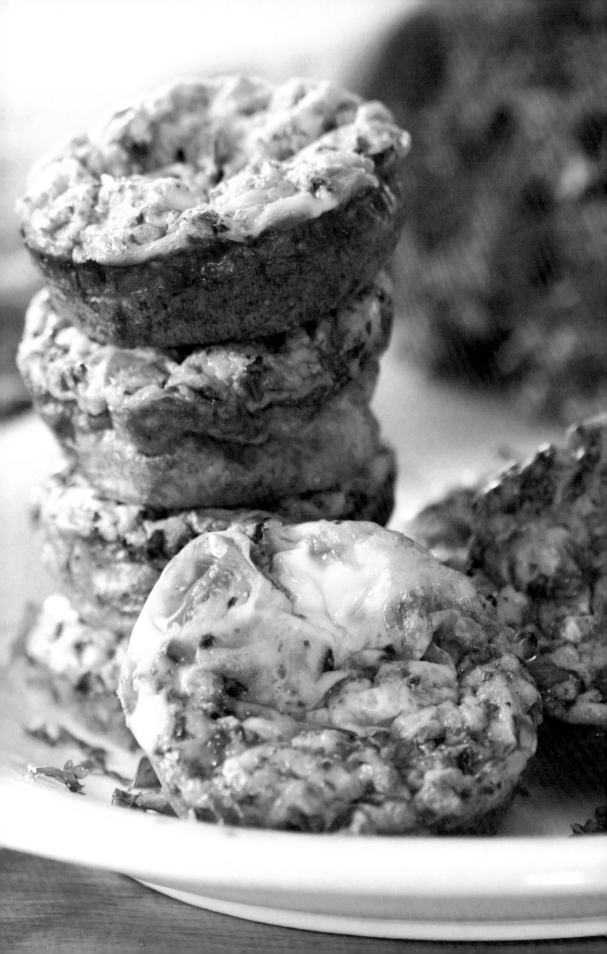

Veggie Egg Cups

INGREDIENTS:

1/4 cup mushrooms

1/4 cup onions

1/4 cup bell pepper

1/4 cup asparagus

1/4 cup spinach

5 eggs

Salt and pepper to taste

OPTIONS:

Add a few dashes of your favorite hot sauce for extra flavor

DIRECTIONS:

Add vegetables to food processor and pulse until chopped very small. If you do not have a food processor, chop by hand.

Place a few drizzles of avocado oil or about a teaspoon of grass-fed butter into a skillet and melt over medium heat. Add chopped vegetables and cook until almost soft.

Allow to cool and add to whisked eggs. Pour mixture into prepared muffin tin. Bake at 350° for 20-25 minutes, or until golden on sides and toothpick runs clean.

• • • • • •

These veggie egg cups are more veggie than eggs. Feel free to change any vegetables or add your favorites; anything will work! They can be made ahead of time and stored in the refrigerator for up to four days or stored in the freezer. If freezing, take out one or two cups and set in refrigerator the night before you plan on eating them, and reheat in whichever way you prefer.

When storing in the refrigerator, it may be helpful to layer the bottom of the container with paper towels to absorb any of the moisture from the vegetables that may sweat out.

BENEFITS OF EGGS:

Vitamin rich eggs are good for the heart, aid in weight management because of their high protein content, and contain oxygenating carotenoids that are good for eye and skin health. They are also rich in choline which has been shown to help with depression and memory related issues.

Prep Time: 5 min.
Total Time: 35 min.
Servings: 8 egg cups

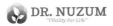

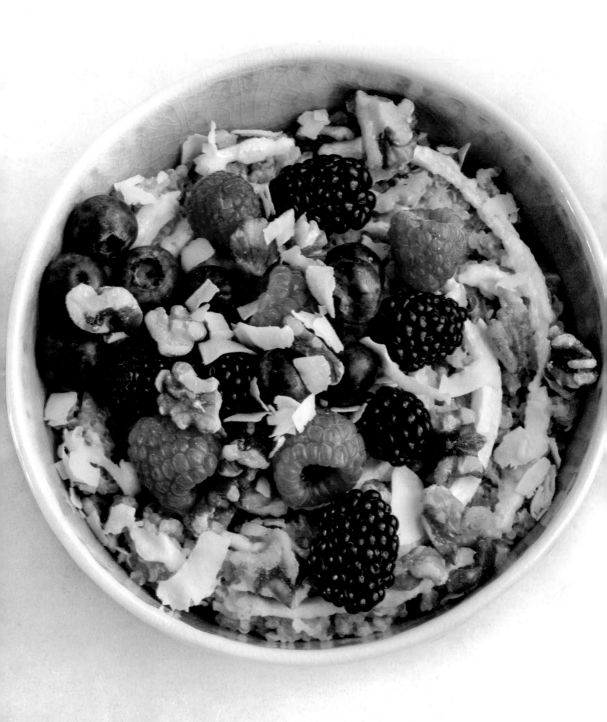

Oat-less Quinoa Oatmeal

INGREDIENTS:

4 cups organic quinoa, rinsed and soaked for 3-6 hours

64 ounces unsweetened coconut or almond milk (2 containers)

1/3 cup pure maple syrup

1/3 cup raw honey

2 teaspoons vanilla

2 teaspoons cinnamon

1/2 teaspoon Himalayan pink salt

DIRECTIONS:

Add all ingredients except one of the 32-ounce containers of nut milk to a large sauce pan. Simmer on medium-low for one hour. Stay with the cereal and stir often. As the liquid cooks down, slowly add your other 32-ounce container of milk. Simmer for ten minutes, stir, add a bit more liquid, and repeat. Cook until liquid is absorbed.

Serve with fresh organic berries, pomegranate seeds, pumpkin seeds, coconut shavings, walnuts, and whipped coconut cream.

———————•••••••———————

Oatmeal is one of those comfort foods that isn't allowed while detoxing, but with this recipe, you'll still have a delicious hot cereal. This version is grain, gluten, and dairy-free and is full of superfoods to help your body detox and heal.

Follow the recipe closely to allow the quinoa to pop and become soft and tender.

BENEFITS OF QUINOA:

Quinoa is technically a seed that is treated like, and eaten similarly to, a grain. It is very high in protein, which makes it a great way for people who are vegan or vegetarian to get adequate protein in their diets. Quinoa also contains quercetin and kaempferol, both flavonoids, that have anti-inflammatory, anti-viral, anti-cancer, and anti-depressant effects in studies.

Prep Time: 1 hour
Serves: 8

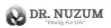

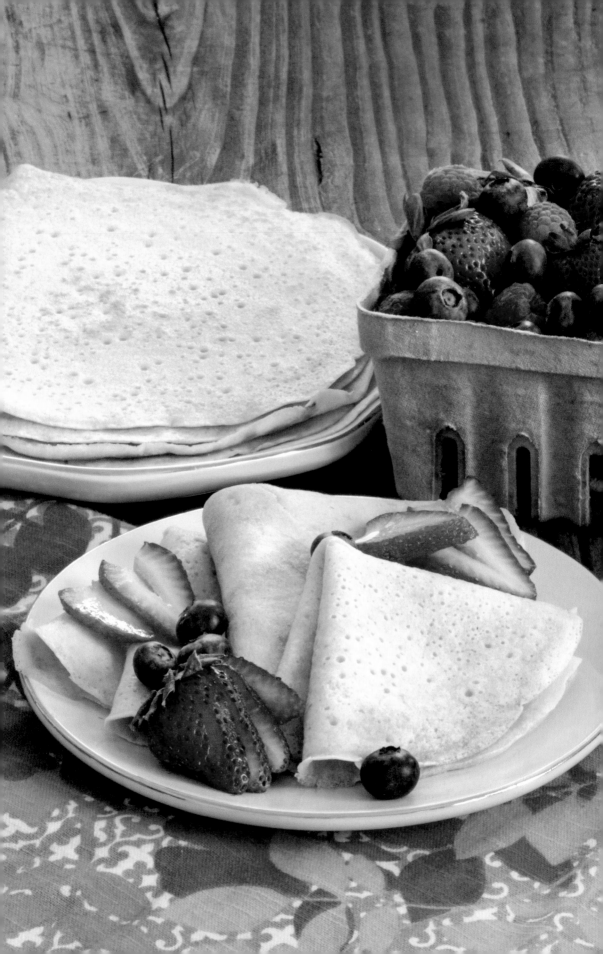

Grain Free Crepes

INGREDIENTS:

1 cup almond flour

1/2 cup tapioca flour or 1/4 arrowroot starch or flour

4 eggs

1 cup almond milk

Pinch of salt

2 tablespoons melted grass-fed butter or coconut oil

OPTIONAL:

1/2 teaspoon vanilla extract

1 tablespoon pure maple syrup, honey, or coconut sugar

DIRECTIONS:

Combine all ingredients in a blender. Mixture should be runny and light yellow color.

Add a teaspoon of coconut oil to a 12 inch pan over medium heat. Once heated, pour about 1/4 cup of the liquid crepe mix to evenly cover the bottom. Wait two to three minutes for the bottom to lightly brown, then flip to cook the other side. You may need to reduce your heat depending on your pan or stove.

Fill with desired berries, coconut cream, or even Greek yogurt—only adding a small amount of yogurt if you aren't on one of the detox protocols.

• • • • •

I have one picky eater in the house and even she approves of these crepes!

Growing up in Mexico, I was the crepe maker in the house for my family. When we went gluten free, and almost all grain free (we still do oats and some rice for the kids), I missed making crepes—a lot. But with this recipe, I don't miss crepes anymore and can still enjoy this lovely treat on a Saturday morning.

BENEFITS OF COCONUT OIL:

Coconut oil is antibacterial, antiviral, and antifungal. It is excellent for helping to fight inflammation, balance hormones, and support a healthy digestive system. It can also help boost energy and metabolism and promotes ketosis. It has been shown to help hypothyroid patients and type 1 and type 2 diabetics.

Prep Time: 10 min.
Makes 12-15 crepes

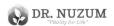

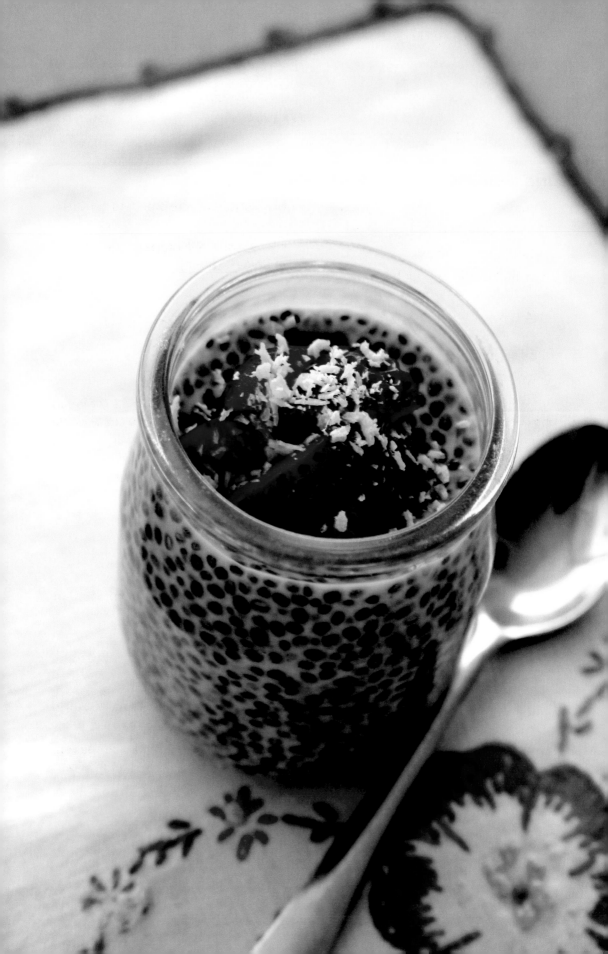

Chia Pudding Jars

INGREDIENTS:

1 cup of chia seeds

4 cups coconut milk

1 tablespoon vanilla

Pinch of Celtic or pink Himalayan sea salt

1/4 cup raw maple syrup or honey

OPTIONS:

May substitute your preferred non-dairy milk

May substitute 5 drops of liquid stevia in place of honey

DIRECTIONS:

Mix all ingredients in a large bowl, then pour into small jars or bowls (or it can stay in a glass bowl and scoop when ready to serve). Stir and mix well to dissolve clumps and refrigerate overnight, or four hours before serving.

• • • • •

This pudding is great topped with unsweetened coconut flakes, cinnamon, or any fresh fruit of your choice.

BENEFITS OF CHIA SEEDS:

Chia seeds are rich in antioxidants and high in fiber, packed with Omega-3 fatty acids for a healthy body and brain as well as being credited with enhancing cognitive performance.

They are a quality source of protein and aid the body in reducing inflammation. They also help to lower bad cholesterol and blood pressure. Chia seeds help to control appetite and balance blood sugar levels.

Prep Time: 5 min.
Serves: 6-8

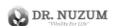

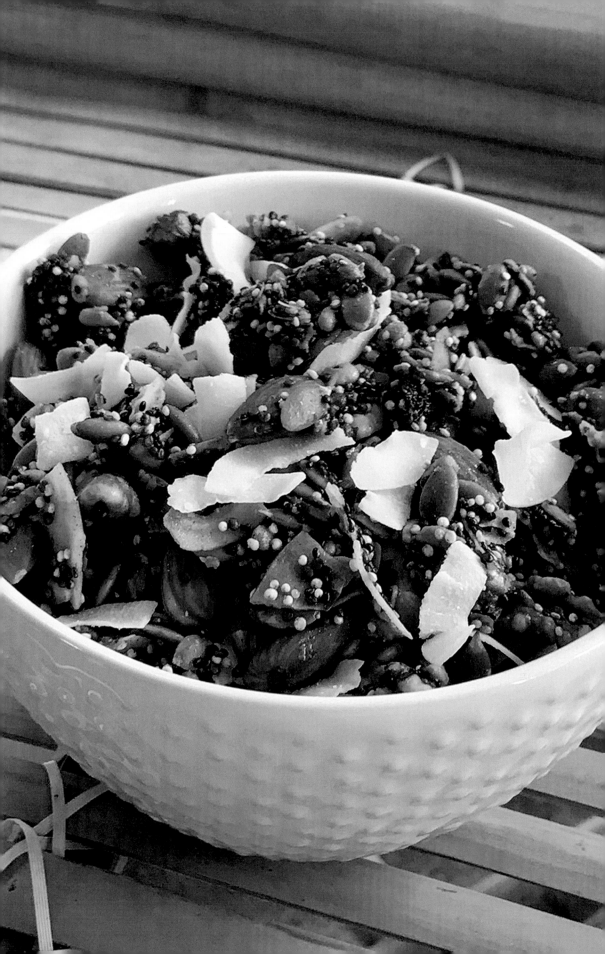

Grain-Free Granola

INGREDIENTS:

2 cups dry quinoa

1/3 cup chia seeds

2 cups pumpkin seeds

2 cups sunflower seeds

1 cup almonds

1 cup walnuts

2 cups unsweetened coconut flakes

1 cup blueberries or cranberries

1/4 cup coconut oil

1/4 cup honey

1 teaspoon cinnamon

3 tablespoons maple syrup

Dash of salt

2 teaspoons real vanilla

DIRECTIONS:

Combine coconut oil, cinnamon, maple syrup, vanilla, and honey in medium pot over low heat. When melted, stir in the rest of the ingredients except fruit, and coat well.

Spread mixture over two cookie sheets lined with parchment paper. Bake at 250° for 30-35 minutes, stirring once halfway through.

Remove from oven and add fruit, mixing well. When cool enough to touch, press the granola tightly together to make bite-size pieces. Store in small bags.

Note: I use chlorine free unbleached parchment baking paper. You can find it at some health food stores or online.

—————●• • • • •●—————

This granola recipe is full of goodness. It's quick and easy to make a large batch and will last up to two weeks if placed in bags. Feel free to mix and match your nuts and dried fruits, just make sure to use organic products.

BENEFITS OF PUMPKIN SEEDS:

Pumpkin seeds are high in many health-supporting nutrients such as magnesium, zinc, manganese, and copper. This zinc-rich seed has been found to support prostate health in men. Other studies suggest pumpkin seeds may help regulate insulin, which can prevent complications experienced by diabetics.

Prep Time: 15 min.
Total Time: 50 min.
Servings: 12-14 cups

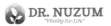

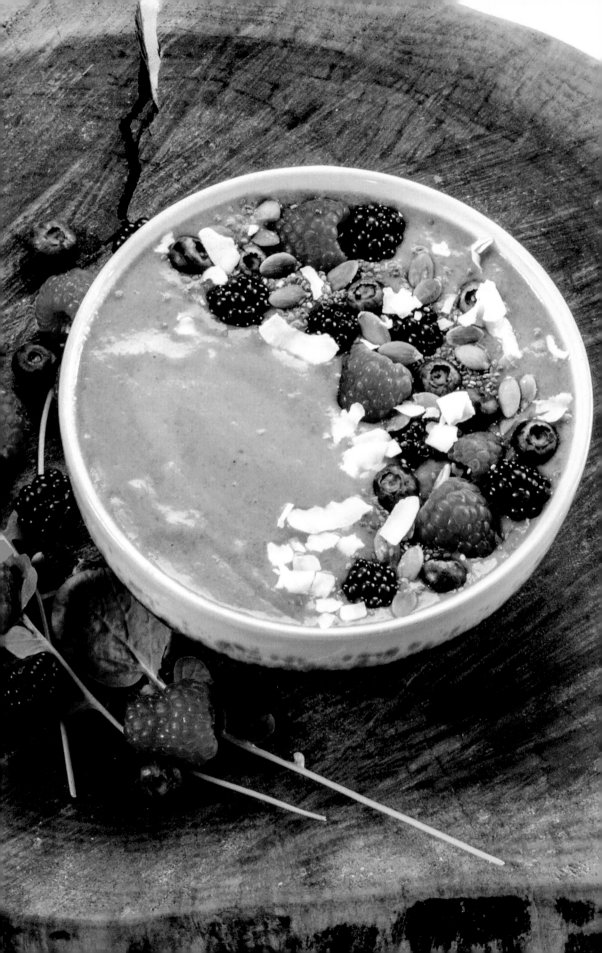

Green Smoothie Fruit Bowl

INGREDIENTS:

2 cups packed spinach

1 cup watercress

1 frozen banana

1/2 cup coconut milk or almond milk

Ice, for thickening

Fresh berries

OPTIONAL:

1/2 teaspoon chia seeds

1 tablespoon pepitas

1/2 tablespoon coconut shavings

DIRECTIONS:

Add spinach, watercress, frozen banana, and coconut milk in a high speed blender.

Add ice to achieve desired thickness.

Add toppings above, or toppings of your choice.

Smoothie bowls are thicker than smoothies that are blended for drinking. They have a yogurt or pudding-like consistency and are meant to be eaten with a spoon.

BENEFITS OF SPINACH:

High in antioxidants and rich in folate, spinach is an anti-inflammatory food and a cancer fighting dark leafy green, rich in vitamins and minerals. Spinach contains vitamin A, which is good for viral infections and the mucous membranes, vitamin C, which is good for connective tissue and a strong immune system, Vitamin E, which is good for anti-oxidizing the fat stored in hormone producing glands and in the brain; and Vitamin K, which enhances vitamin D absorption. Spinach is also rich in calcium which is good for the teeth and bones, and potassium, which is good for the heart and kidneys. It is also high in protein, fiber, and folate, which is important for gene replication.

Prep Time: 10 min.
Serves: 1

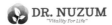

Snacks, Dips & Sauces

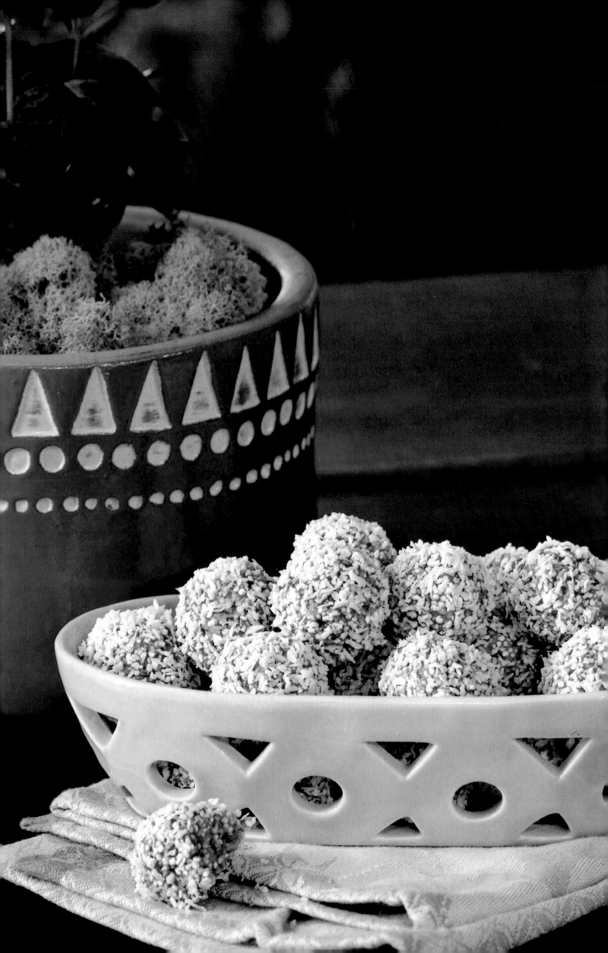

No-Bake Energy Bites

INGREDIENTS:

1/3 cup pecans, finely chopped

1/3 cup cashews, finely chopped

1/3 cup almonds, finely chopped

1/2 cup almond butter

1/3 cup coconut oil

2/3 unsweetened coconut flakes

1/2 cup ground flaxseed

1 tablespoon chia seeds

1 teaspoon vanilla extract

2 tablespoons honey (raw or unfiltered)

1/4 teaspoon Himalayan pink salt

DIRECTIONS:

Mix well in a bowl until all ingredients are thoroughly combined. Put mixture in refrigerator for thirty minutes to one hour, to better form balls. With your hands, form mixture into one inch balls and roll them in coconut flakes. Store in refrigerator. Eat one to three balls for a snack.

There will be days during Dr. Nuzum's 2-Week Detox, or any day really, where you may feel you need more calories and protein. These energy bites are great for those moments and great for on-the-go.

BENEFITS OF ALMONDS:

Almonds are a great source of antioxidants, which are largely concentrated in their brown skin. These antioxidants protect against oxidative stress, which can damage molecules in cells and contribute to diseases like cancer. Its high levels of vitamin E also protect cell membranes from damage, as well as lower risk for heart disease, cancer, and Alzheimer's disease.

Prep Time: 10 min.
Total Time: 50 min.
Makes 12-18 bites

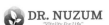

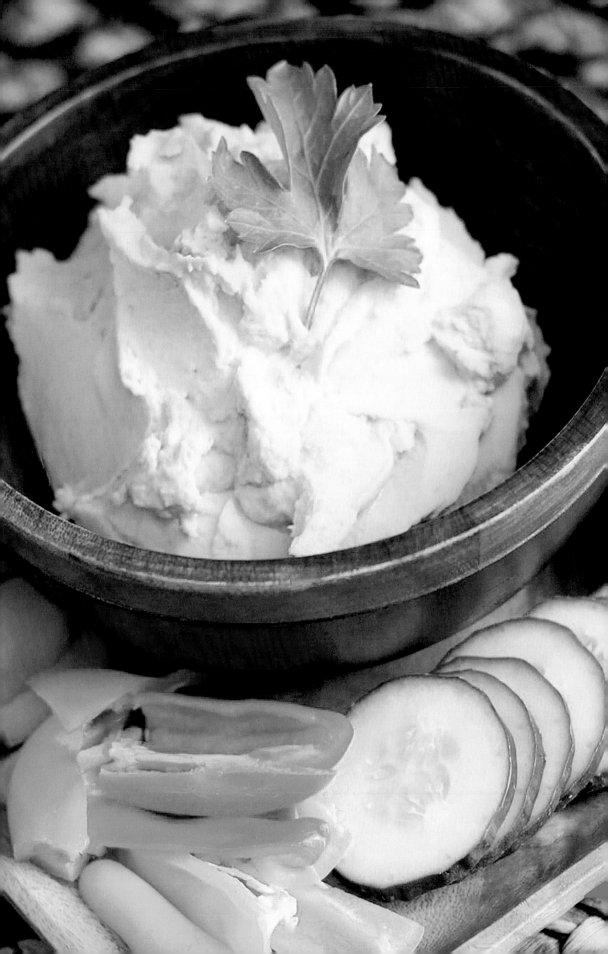

Classic Hummus

INGREDIENTS:

3 cups cooked garbanzo beans (also called chickpeas)

2 tablespoons tahini

4 tablespoons olive oil

1 large garlic clove

1/8 teaspoon cumin powder

3-5 tablespoons filtered water

1/2 to 1 whole lemon, juiced

1/2 teaspoon Himalayan pink salt

DIRECTIONS:

Combine all ingredients in a food processor or a high speed blender and blend until smooth.

Adjust salt and lemon to your desired taste.

Adjust water according to texture.

Serve with fresh cut vegetables or use as a spread.

—————————•••••—————————

If you cook extra garbanzo beans, you can add some to your favorite salad or soup; they make an excellent addition.

BENEFITS OF GARBANZO BEANS:

Garbanzo beans help keep the digestive system free from harmful bacteria and pathogens as well as toxic build up. This makes them an anti-inflammatory food and cancer fighter. They are a good source of plant based protein and soluble fiber, which promotes a healthy digestive system. Chickpeas help to stabilize blood sugar levels and help to reduce cravings. They are also known to balance unhealthy cholesterol. Chickpeas are high in Zinc, making this bean a great immune system booster. They are a great source of folate (vitamin B9), which is important for making healthy new cells. They are also known for their ability to reduce symptoms of PMS because of the magnesium, manganese, and vitamin B6.

> Prep Time: 10 min.
> Serves: 4

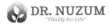

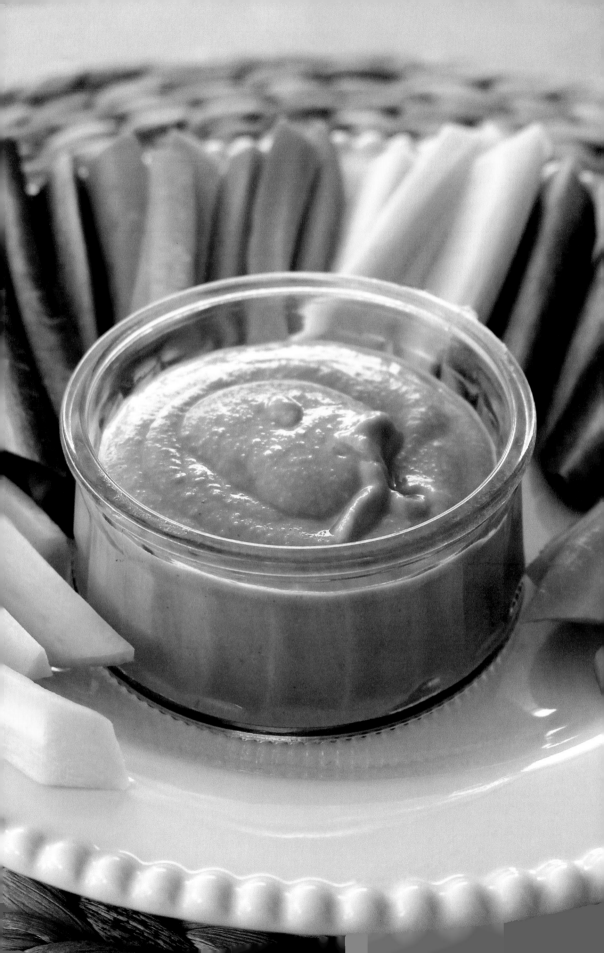

Cilantro Hummus

INGREDIENTS:

2 cups fully cooked chickpeas, also called garbanzo beans

1/4 cup fresh lemon or lime juice

1 large garlic clove (or half a clove, depending on how much you like garlic)

2 tablespoons cold pressed organic olive oil

Bunch of cilantro (approximately 1 1/2 cups)

1/4 to 1/2 teaspoon of pink Himalayan, Celtic, or sea salt (adjust as desired)

1/4 teaspoon of dried organic turmeric powder (optional)

2 to 3 teaspoon water

Dash of ground pepper for serving

DIRECTIONS:

Soak the chickpeas the day before. Boil in water for one to two hours, adding salt in the last thirty minutes of boil. You can also use a slow cooker.

Blend all ingredients in a blender or food processor until smooth, adjusting water for consistency.

Be careful to not overdo it on salt—your chickpeas may have enough salt from when they were boiling.

● ● ● ● ● ●

This Hummus makes a great dip for fresh veggies anytime. Make an all veggie hummus lettuce wrap with this spread, adding sliced carrots and cucumbers.

BENEFITS OF CILANTRO:

Cilantro is a fresh herb that has been used in cooking for thousands of years. Extracts from the leaf can protect skin against damage from ultra violet radiation. Its leaves also contain dodecanal, which has an antibacterial affect against salmonella. Finally, cilantro is a natural chelator that can help combat toxicity from lead and other heavy metals.

Prep Time: 10 min.
Serves: 4-6

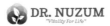

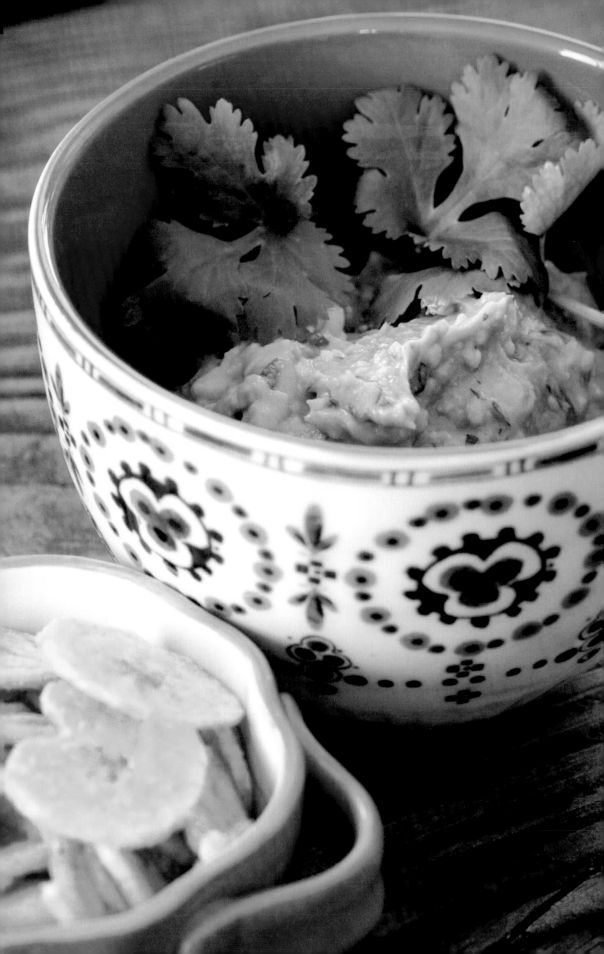

Classic Guacamole

INGREDIENTS:

3 ripe avocados, halved, seeded, and peeled

1/2 tablespoon lime juice

1/2 teaspoon Himalayan pink salt

1/2 medium red onion, diced

1/2 jalapeño pepper, seeded, and minced

2 Roma tomatoes, seeded and diced

2 tablespoons cilantro, finely chopped

1 clove garlic, minced

DIRECTIONS:

Add scooped avocado, lime juice, and salt to a large bowl. Mash together with fork until avocado achieves the preferred texture.

Fold in remaining ingredients and let sit for up to an hour.

Serve with plantain chips.

TIP:

You can also simplify this recipe by mashing avocados with salt, garlic and onion powders, and cayenne pepper to taste.

It is completely normal to want to eat things that are familiar to us. This version of "chips and guac" hits the spot and and also helps relieve the feeling of being excluded from party activities that involve snack foods—just remember to bring your own plantain chips! There is zero guilt with this snack.

BENEFITS OF AVOCADOS:

Some of the wonderful things avocados provide are heart-healthy mono-unsaturated fatty acids, many vitamins, more potassium than bananas, and plenty of fiber. So, go ahead and dip that chip!

Prep Time: 10 min.
Serves: 4

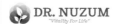

Strawberry Mint Pico

INGREDIENTS:

1/2 cucumber, chopped

2 cups strawberries, chopped

1/2 cup mango, chopped

1 lime, juiced

1 tablespoon honey

Dash pink Himalayan salt

1/8 cup fresh mint, chopped

DIRECTIONS:

Combine all ingredients in a bowl and stir well. This dish is simple to prepare, beautiful, and full of flavors that kids love.

———————— • • • • • ————————

This is a fun, sweet, minty-limey salsa. It's great to eat by itself, to put on top of grilled chicken, or to top a salad.

Prep Time: 10 min.
Serves: 2-4

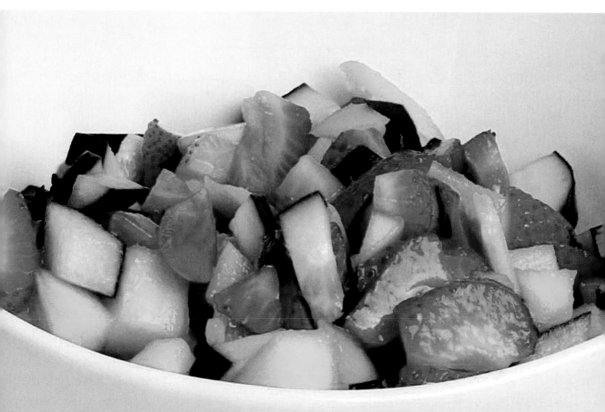

Strawberry Pineapple Salsa

INGREDIENTS:

1/2 organic pineapple, chopped in small pieces

1 cup organic chopped strawberries

1/4 habanero chili pepper, chopped very fine

2 whole green onions, chopped fine (green and white parts)

1/2 cup organic cilantro, chopped fine

1/2 large lemon, zested and juiced

1 tablespoon organic avocado oil or cold-pressed, extra-virgin olive oil

2 tablespoons of organic apple cider vinegar

Salt and pepper to taste

DIRECTIONS:

Add ingredients to medium bowl and mix well. Marinate for one to two hours in refrigerator.

· · · · ·

While in the refrigerator, the fruit will start to break down and juices will release from the fruit. You may need to add a little honey if the fruit is not ripe or sweet enough. This salsa goes very well with the Grilled Chicken Tacos on page 213.

BENEFITS OF STRAWBERRIES:

Strawberries are high in antioxidants, which make them a great detox food that helps protect your organs. They are particularly high in vitamin C, folate, potassium, manganese, dietary fiber, and magnesium. These little red powerhouses are great for boosting the immune system, maintaining normal blood pressure, reducing risk of arthritis and cancer, and helping to prevent heart disease.

Prep Time: 15 min.
Serves: 2-4

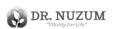

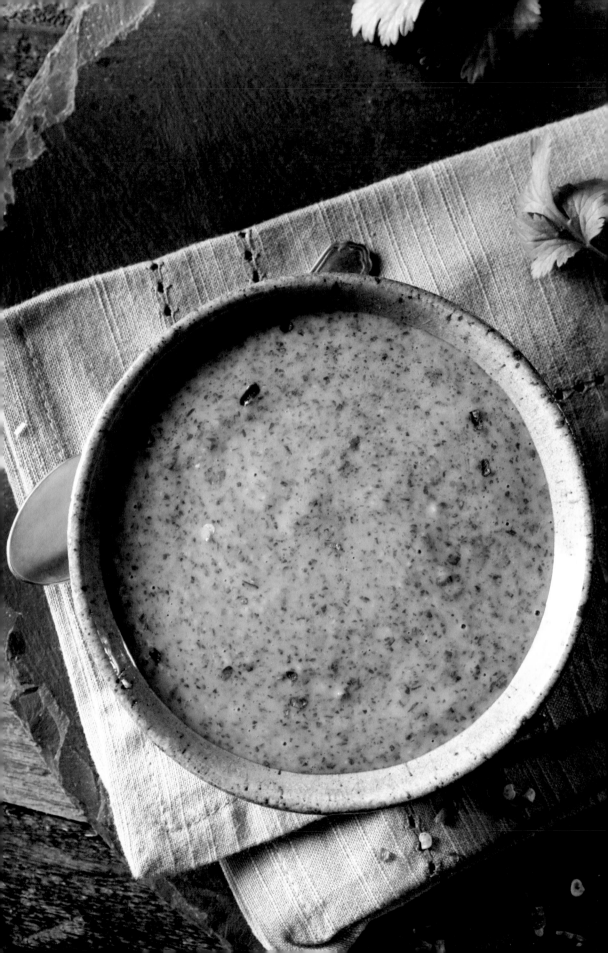

Chimichurri Sauce

INGREDIENTS:

1 bunch Italian parsley (about 2 cups)

1/2 cup olive oil

2-3 garlic cloves

1/4 cup water

1 tablespoon organic nutritional yeast (non-fortified, without MSG)

OPTIONS:

1/2 teaspoon Himalayan pink salt

Ground pepper to taste

A few drops of fresh lemon juice

Spice up the sauce some by adding red pepper flakes to taste

DIRECTIONS:

Combine all ingredients in a blender and blend until smooth. Salt to taste.

This sauce stores well in the refrigerator, lasting five to seven days.

• • • • •

Chimichurri is a staple of Argentinian cuisine and is a detox food for sure, with garlic, parsley, and olive oil. It is usually eaten on steak, but since there are no steak recipes here, feel free to use it on many different dishes. I promise, you will love this green flavor bomb! You can add a tablespoon to a vegetable soup, use it as a marinade for vegetables or chicken, or add it to one of my other recipes like the Quinoa Vegetable Bowl on page 221.

BENEFITS OF PARSLEY:

Parsley is a super green food that detoxifies both the kidneys and the liver. It reduces toxic build up in the kidneys, which can lead to kidney stones. It also enhances the body's pH.

Prep Time: 5 min.
Serves: 4-6

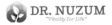

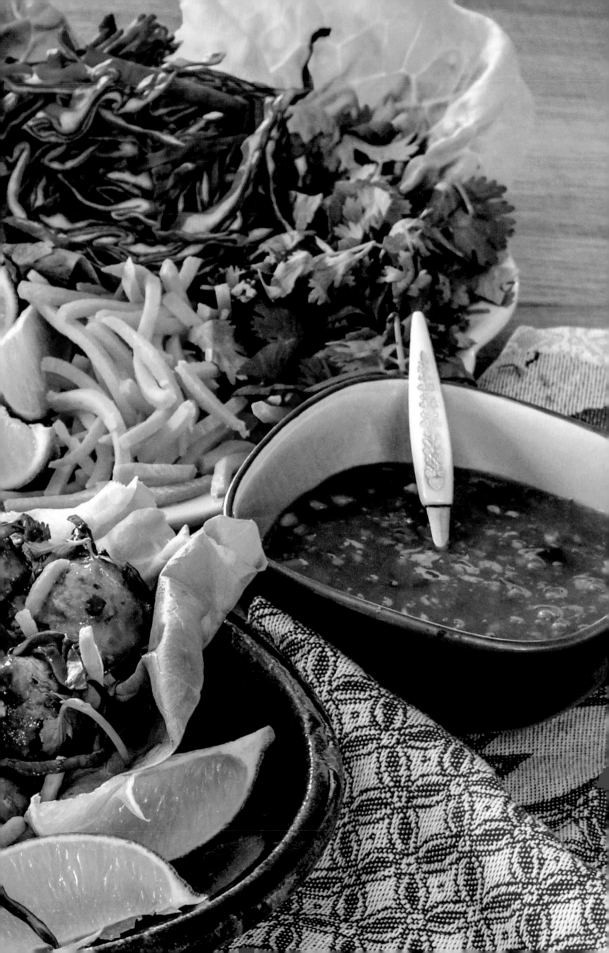

Asian Sauce

INGREDIENTS:

1 cup fresh squeezed orange juice

2 limes, juiced

1/4 cup coconut aminos

1/2 cup water

3 cloves garlic, minced

1 tablespoon ginger, finely minced

3 tablespoons arrowroot powder

Additional 1/4 cup water

DIRECTIONS:

Mix arrowroot powder and 1/4 cup water with whisk until smooth in small bowl. Set aside until later.

Place remaining ingredients in medium sauce pan. Bring to a boil then turn down to medium-low heat. Let simmer for 20 minutes, stirring occasionally. After the sauce has simmered for 20 minutes, slowly whisk in arrowroot mixture and let cook for 5 more minutes to slightly thicken.

● • • • • ●

This sauce is great with any Asian themed dish, but goes particularly well with the Asian Meatball Lettuce Wraps on page 225.

BENEFITS OF GARLIC:

Garlic contains allicin, a sulphur-containing compound that has anti-bacterial and anti-fungal properties. This natural antibiotic can help flush toxins from the digestive system. To maximize the benefits of raw garlic, bite a clove to crush it between your back teeth, then swallow whole with water.

Total Time: 30 min.
Makes 2 1/2 cups

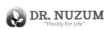

Soups

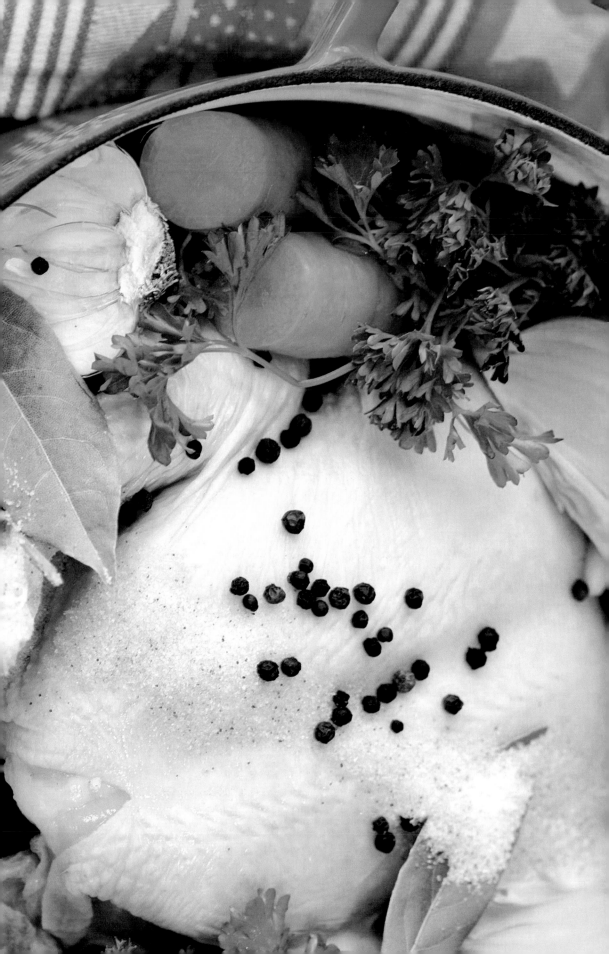

Chicken Broth

INGREDIENTS:

1 whole organic chicken or carcass

2 celery stalks, cut in half

2 large carrots, cut in half

1 yellow onion, unpeeled, cut into quarters

1 garlic head, unpeeled, cut in half

1 bunch of parsley

2 bay leaves

2 tablespoons Himalayan pink salt

1 teaspoon whole peppercorns

1 tablespoon raw apple cider vinegar

DIRECTIONS:

Put all ingredients into a stock pot or Dutch oven. Add filtered or reverse osmosis water until chicken is covered. Let sit for 30 minutes, then bring to a simmer on medium-low heat. Skim off any foam at the top, turn the heat to low and allow to simmer with the lid ajar for 8-24 hours. Add water as liquid evaporates.

Once cooled, strain broth and discard vegetables, herbs, and peppercorns. Set chicken aside and use in soups, salads, or however else you would like. Store broth in refrigerator for up to one week, or in the back of the freezer for up to six months.

• • • • •

Homemade chicken broth is a game changer. Once you start making homemade broth, you won't go back to store-bought. Don't be intimidated by this, it is so simple to make!

BENEFITS OF CHICKEN BROTH:

Besides the fact that homemade chicken broth is so much tastier than store-bought, it is also incredibly healing for the body. Store-bought broths often have ingredients like MSG and additives that aren't beneficial to you and they also lack gelatin—one of the most wonderful things about broth. Gelatin has many benefits—one of them is its healing power on your digestive system and stomach lining. It contains trace minerals and amino acids that actually detoxify the body.

Prep Time: 15 min.
Total Time: 8-24 hours
Servings: 6-8

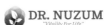

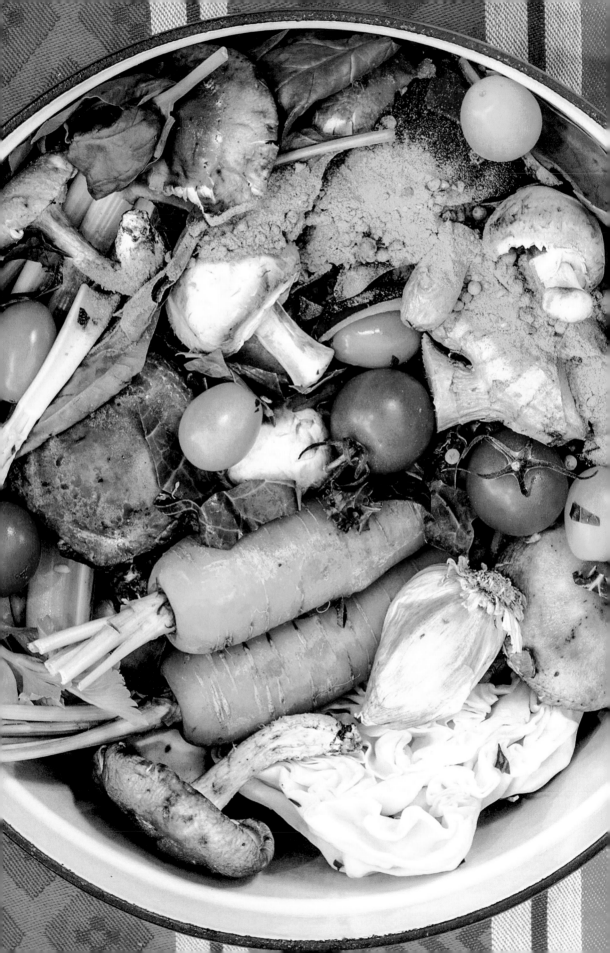

Gut Healing Vegetable Broth

INGREDIENTS:

12 cups filtered water

1 tablespoon avocado oil

1 red onion, cut in 4 pieces (with skin)

1 large garlic bulb, smashed with skin

1 knuckle ginger, chopped with skin

1 cup kale

1 cup spinach

1 tablespoon raw apple cider vinegar

1/2 cup parsley, finely chopped

3 or 4 chopped vegetables with skin (carrots, cabbage, celery, mushrooms)

1/2 cup dried shiitake mushrooms (or fresh mushrooms)

1 bunch cherry tomatoes

Spices:

1 tablespoon peppercorns

2 tablespoons ground or fresh turmeric

2 tablespoons coconut aminos

1 teaspoon dried coriander or a bunch of fresh coriander (optional)

2-3 tablespoons pink Himalayan salt, adjust to taste

DIRECTIONS:

Combine all ingredients in a large pot. Bring to a gentle boil then simmer for about an hour with the lid on medium-low heat. Drain liquid into a storage container, straining out vegetables. Top remaining vegetables with your favorite fresh herbs and serve hot.

Note: I left the carrots and other veggies whole for photography purposes, but I cut them into pieces at the time of serving. Dice veggies before adding to the pot to create a vegetable soup or to make bite size portions.

• • • • •

This broth freezes well. You will have enough for the whole family or for the 3-Day Liquid Detox program on page 98. This can also be made in a slow cooker overnight or through the day.

BENEFITS OF SHIITAKE MUSHROOMS:

Shiitake mushrooms benefit the body in many ways. One of the most healing compounds found in Shiitake is lentinan, which can heal chromosome damage caused by allopathic treatments for cancer. This mushroom also contains all eight essential amino acids, benefits bone-building, improves digestion, and reduces food allergies.

Prep Time: 15 min.
Total Time: 90 min.
Servings: 6-8

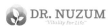

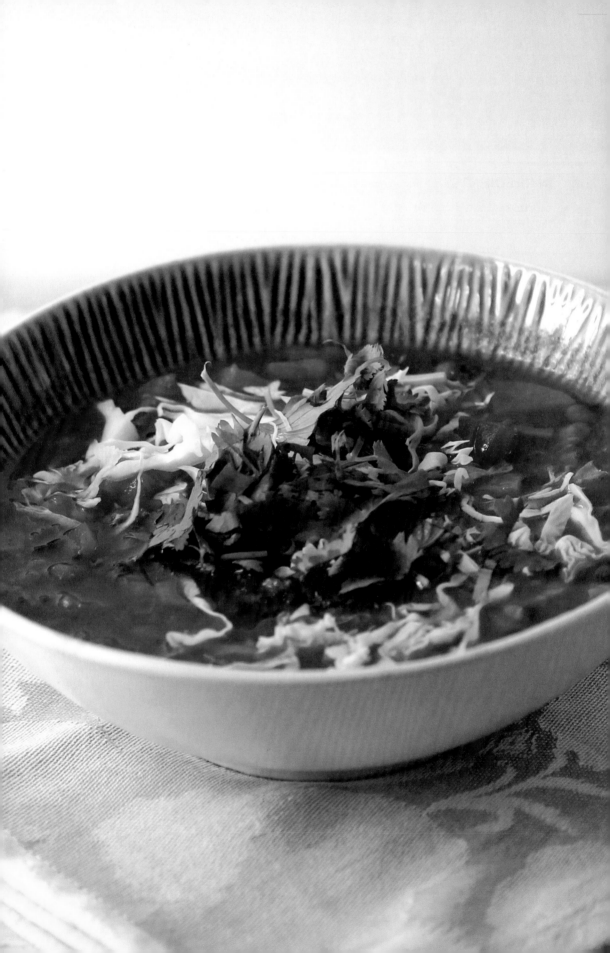

Veggie Lentil Soup

INGREDIENTS:

2 cups soaked lentils (soak the night before)

2 cups water

1 large sweet potato, chopped

2 cups broccoli florets

Tomato Base:

1/2 onion, chopped

1 large tomato, chopped

4 celery stalks, finely chopped

Bunch cilantro, chopped (save some for the topping)

1 large clove of garlic, minced (and an extra one for the broth)

In the blender:

3 large tomatoes

6 cups water

1/4 medium onion

Spices:

1/2 teaspoon cumin powder

1/4 teaspoon ginger powder

1/4 teaspoon cinnamon powder

2 teaspoons salt

1/4 teaspoon pepper

DIRECTIONS:

Add tomato base to pot with the sautéed vegetables, then add soaked lentils, chopped vegetables, spices, and the two extra cups of water. Add more or less water to adjust the thickness of soup. Bring to medium heat for 10 minutes, then lower heat and keep on low for the next 30-35 minutes.

Top with chopped cabbage and cilantro or avocado.

———————— • • • • • • ————————

This is one of my family's favorite soups; my kids absolutely love it! It is one of those feel good, tummy-warming soups that is also delicious as a leftover—great for when you are doing the 2-Week Detox program or any time.

BENEFITS OF LENTILS:

Lentils are a great choice for weight loss because of their low fat, high nutrition, energy boosting, and blood sugar regulating effects. One cup of lentils provides 18 grams of high plant-based protein. One of the best types of plant based protein (with a low starch content), lentils are rich in potassium, magnesium, folate, calcium, zinc, niacin, iron, and vitamin K. They are one of the easier beans for the body to digest and have a very low impact on blood sugar compared to refined grains.

Total Time: 40 min.
Serves: 6-8

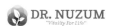

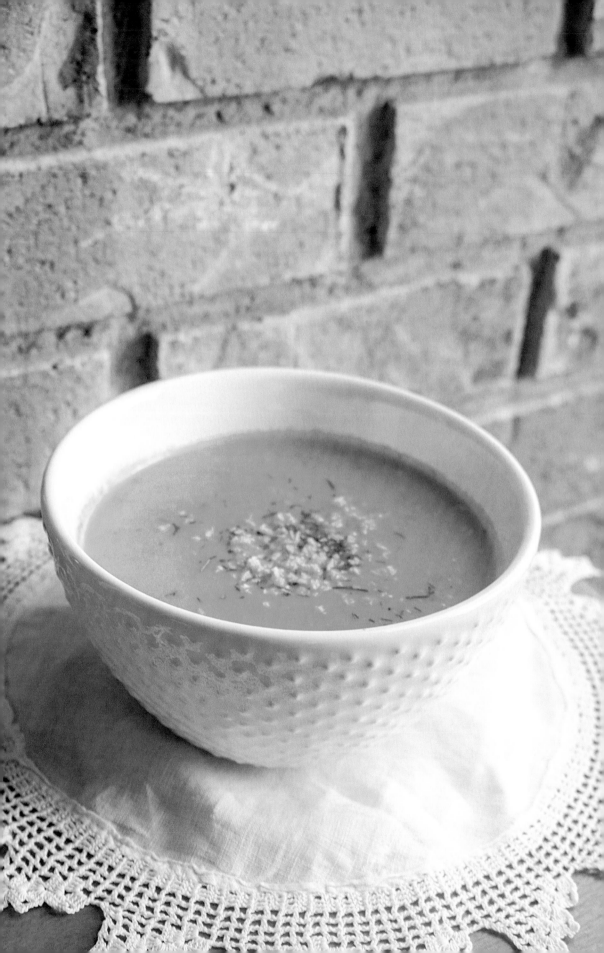

Carrot-Ginger Soup

INGREDIENTS:

1 small yellow onion, diced

3 tablespoons avocado oil

2 celery stalks, chopped

1 garlic clove, minced

1/2 teaspoon cumin

1/2 teaspoon cinnamon

1 small piece of fresh ginger (about 1 inch), peeled and grated

1 small piece of fresh turmeric root (about 1 inch), peeled and grated

8 medium sized carrots, cut into pieces

4 cups of water (or chicken broth)

1 teaspoon white pepper

1 1/2 teaspoons salt

OPTIONS:

1/2 teaspoon powdered ginger

May use 1/2 teaspoon turmeric powder to replace the turmeric root

May add coconut aminos for taste

DIRECTIONS:

Saute onions and celery in large pot with avocado oil on medium to low heat.

Once onions and celery begin to turn translucent, add grated ginger, minced garlic, cumin, cinnamon, ginger powder, and turmeric. Stir constantly on medium heat for 1-2 minutes. Add carrots and liquid, then bring to a gentle boil. Cover and let simmer on low heat for about 20 minutes, or until carrots become soft.

Once carrots are fully cooked, let the stock cool, then blend in a high-speed blender. Add more liquid if necessary to achieve desired texture. Once blended, return to pot, and season with salt and pepper to taste. Top with coconut flakes and serve hot.

NOTE: Keep in mind, ginger can make food quite spicy.

BENEFITS OF CARROTS:

Rich in vitamin A, carrots are well known for helping maintain good eyesight. Eating carrots can also help lower blood sugar levels and regulate insulin levels. Beta-carotene and high fiber content are also known to decrease chances of colon, lung, and breast cancer.

Total Time: 40 min.
Serves: 4-6

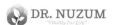

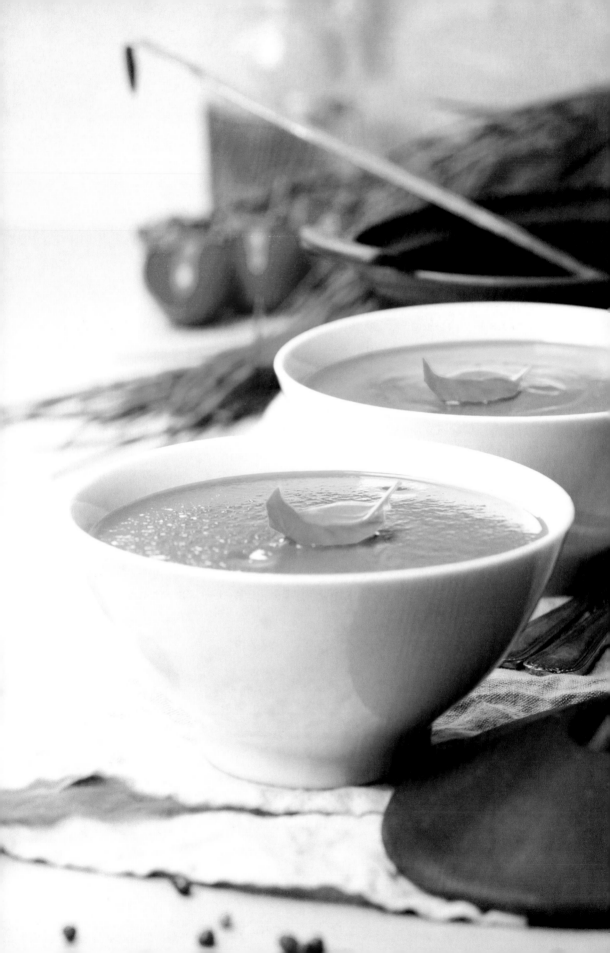

Cream of Tomato

INGREDIENTS:

6 large fresh tomatoes, chopped

3 stalks celery, chopped

1 whole yellow onion, chopped

1/2 yellow or red pepper, chopped

1 large carrot, finely chopped

3 cloves of garlic, finely chopped

1 cup fresh basil leaves, chopped

3 cups vegetable stock

3 cups water

1 teaspoon salt

1 teaspoon pepper

2 tablespoons honey

12 ounces coconut milk (preferably not from a can)

DIRECTIONS:

Bring all ingredients to boil in medium sauce pan, cooking vegetables until tender, then turn heat down to simmer for 30 minutes. Remove from heat to let cool for 10-15 minutes.

Pour warm mixture into blender and blend until smooth. Start on low and build speed to avoid splashing. Cover with kitchen towel to avoid burns. Depending on the size of your blender, you might have to process the soup in two batches.

Pour soup back in the pan and add the coconut milk and honey. Stir well. Reheat soup to serving temperature and add salt to desired taste.

Garnish with a bit of hot pepper flakes, fresh ground pepper, and a basil leaf.

Note: Allow soup to cool before blending because adding hot liquid to plastic can release unwanted toxins.

• • • • •

This comforting soup is rich and creamy, but also incredibly good for you. If using a Vitamix to blend soup, the soup will turn out completely smooth. If using another type of blender, the soup may have a bit more texture. The abundance of vegetables in this soup is really what gives it all of its flavor, nutrients, and health benefits.

BENEFITS OF TOMATOES:

Tomatoes have vitamin C, A, K, folate, potassium, thiamin, niacin, magnesium, vitamin B6, phosphorus, copper, and incredibly important fiber. Tomatoes contain alpha and beta carotene, lutein, and finally, lycopene—considered the highest in antioxidant activity of the four major carotenoids.

Total Time: 45 min.
Serves: 4

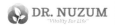

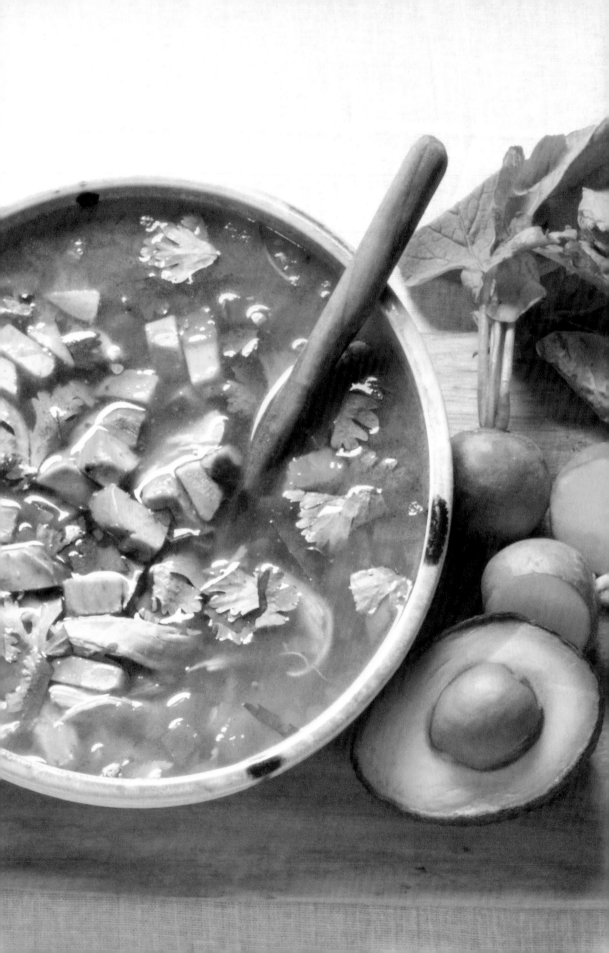

Chicken Chile Verde

INGREDIENTS:

2 cups cooked chicken meat, chopped or shredded

3 tablespoons avocado oil

1 large white onion, chopped

1/2 yellow pepper, finely chopped

1 package mild, roasted green chiles, thawed (look for Select New Mexico brand, 24-ounce bag of roasted green chiles in freezer section by frozen vegetables)

3 cloves garlic, minced

1 teaspoon cumin

1 teaspoon chili powder

1 teaspoon salt

1/2 teaspoon pepper

6 cups chicken bone broth (see recipe or use organic store bought bone broth)

2 cups water

1 cup water

3 tablespoons arrowroot

Bunch cilantro, chopped for topping

2 ripe avocados, chopped for topping

DIRECTIONS:

Heat oil in a large stock pot, then add chopped onions, yellow pepper, garlic, spices, and salt and pepper. Sauté for 10 minutes. Add thawed green chiles and chicken meat and stir well. Add bone broth and two cups water and stir. Let simmer for 30 minutes on medium heat. Add salt to taste. Mix one cup water and arrowroot in small bowl and stir until smooth. Whisk in thickening mixture after soup has simmered 30 minutes. Let cook another 10 minutes before serving. Top each bowl of soup with fresh chopped cilantro and avocado.

• • • • •

This spicy chicken green soup makes for a wonderful comfort food. It's perfect in a big bowl topped with fresh chopped cilantro and avocado and makes for a great enchilada sauce.

BENEFITS OF GREEN CHILES:

Green chiles are a rich source of vitamin C, B6, copper, iron, potassium, phyto-nutrients like Carotene-B, Carotene-A, Cryptoxanthin-B, and Lutein-zeaxanthin. Chiles help with bone care, skin care, digestion, eye care, delay aging, and they taste amazing! Adding a bit of heat and spice to your diet takes the boring out of eating healthy.

Total Time: 50 min.
Serves: 6

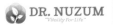

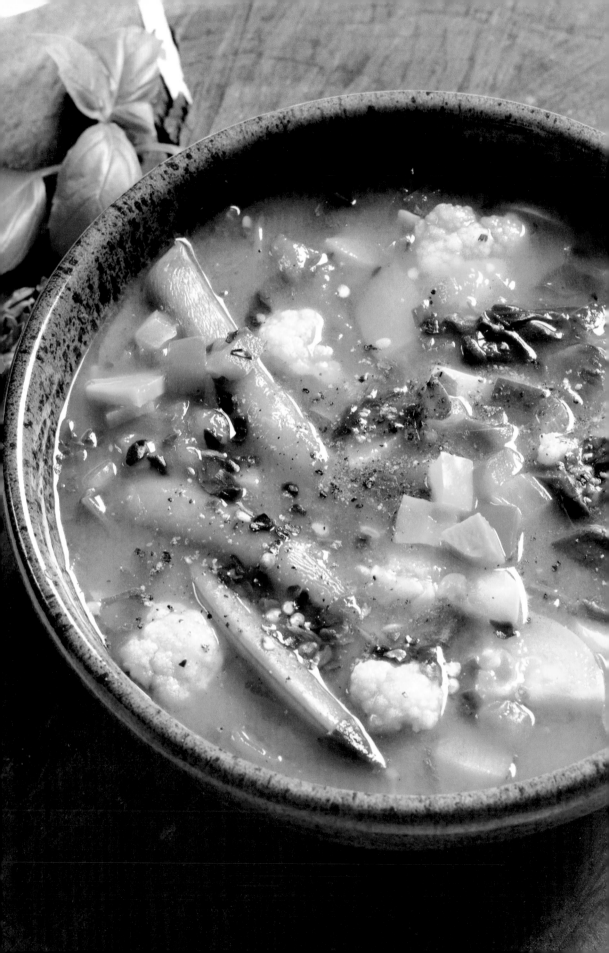

Detox Soup

INGREDIENTS:

6 cups homemade veggie stock

3 large tomatoes, chopped

3 celery stalks, chopped

3 carrots, chopped

1 large onion, chopped

2 tablespoons fresh ginger, grated

2 green chilies roasted, skinned and chopped

1 red or yellow bell pepper, chopped

1 yellow squash, chopped

1 zucchini, chopped

1 cup cauliflower florets, chopped

1 cup Swiss chard, chopped

1 cup fresh snow or snap peas in shell, chopped

1 cup baby spinach

1 lemon, zested and juiced

4 tablespoons fresh parsley, finely chopped

3 tablespoons fresh basil leaves, finely chopped

3 tablespoons avocado oil

1 1/2 teaspoons pink Himalayan salt

1 teaspoon pepper

DIRECTIONS:

Heat oil in large stock pot until very hot. Add celery, carrots, onions, tomatoes, roasted chiles, yellow squash, zucchini, and salt and pepper. Sauté for 10 minutes on high heat.

Add vegetable stock and reduce heat to simmer for 30 minutes or until vegetables are tender. Try not to overcook to retain freshness.

Add cauliflower the last 10 minutes of cooking, then add your snow peas and Swiss chard the last 5 minutes.

Shut off heat and add spinach, fresh herbs, lemon zest and juice. Stir and add salt to taste.

Finish soup with fresh ground pepper, or a pinch of red pepper flakes.

• • • • •

This soup is rich and flavorful. Use homemade vegetable stock from page 181. Finishing the soup with fresh baby spinach, lemon zest, lemon juice, and fresh herbs makes it taste fresh and light. This soup freezes well for up to 6 months.

BENEFITS OF LEMON:

The various acids in lemons, including ascorbic acid (vitamin C), stimulate enzyme production in the digestive tract as well as improve the liver's detoxification.

Total Time: 45 min.
Serves: 6-8

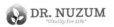

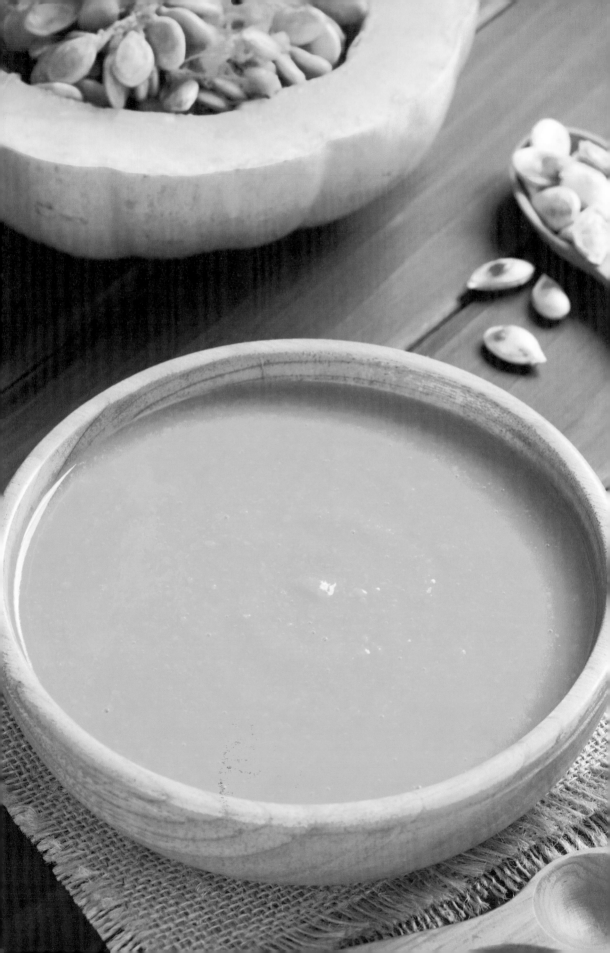

Pumpkin Soup

INGREDIENTS:

1 box pureed pumpkin (approximately 12 to 18 ounces)

1 large sweet potato, peeled and chopped into small pieces

1 large onion, chopped

3 carrots, chopped

5 cups homemade vegetable stock (see vegetable broth recipe on page 181)

1 box (11 ounces) coconut milk

1/2 teaspoon cinnamon

1/2 teaspoon nutmeg

1 teaspoon salt

1/2 teaspoon pepper

1/2 teaspoon dried thyme

2 tablespoons avocado oil

2 teaspoons honey

DIRECTIONS:

Add avocado oil, onions, carrots, and sweet potato to stock pot. Sauté on medium-high heat for 8-10 minutes. Season with salt and pepper.

Add thyme, cinnamon, and nutmeg. Simmer 3 more minutes, then add vegetable stock. Simmer on medium heat for 20-30 minutes, or until vegetables are tender.

Let cool for 5-10 minutes, then add soup to high-speed blender to puree. If the container for your blender is glass, you could blend while hot. Be very careful when blending hot liquids.

Pour soup back in pot to reheat and add coconut milk and honey.

Serve and garnish with a bit of cinnamon and nutmeg in each each bowl.

● ● ● ● ●

This rich and creamy soup will soon be one of your favorites. Adding a sweet potato and carrots adds a depth of flavor that pumpkin alone cannot do. It also adds more nutrition to your soup! This soup comes together quickly and the color and flavor of the soup is rich and warm – perfect for those chilly fall evenings.

BENEFITS OF PUMPKIN:

Pumpkin is full of potassium, magnesium, zinc , vitamin C, and is an incredibly rich source of vitamin A. Pumpkin is excellent for diabetics as it helps regulate blood sugar, and its high fiber and high carotenoid content are wonderful for the heart.

Total Time: 50 min.
Serves: 4

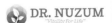

Salads

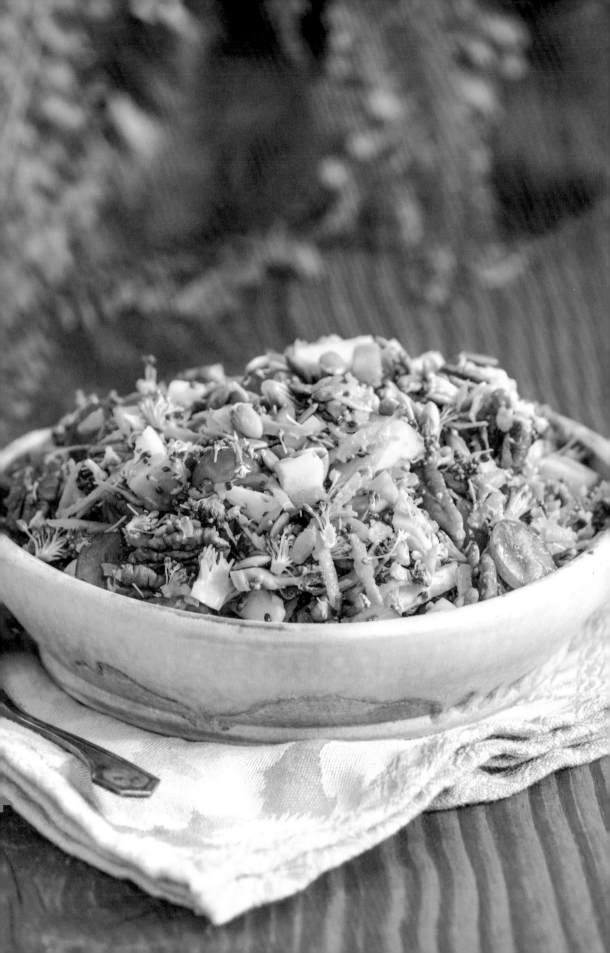

Crunchy Broccoli Salad

INGREDIENTS:

2 cups broccoli, finely chopped

1/2 cup halved grapes

1 cup soaked pecans

1 tablespoon pumpkin seeds, soaked

1/2 apple, chopped

1 tablespoon avocado oil

1 teaspoon apple cider vinegar

1 carrot, shredded

1 1/2 tablespoon honey

1 lemon, juiced

Add salt to taste

DIRECTIONS:

Chop broccoli florets into small pieces so they blend in well with the fruit and seeds.

Combine all ingredients in a large bowl and allow the flavors to incorporate. The flavors improve after a few hours of soaking in the lemon juice and honey.

This salad stores well in the refrigerator.

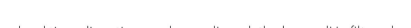

If you have a hard time digesting raw broccoli, soak the broccoli in filtered water and apple cider vinegar for 30 minutes, or steam the broccoli.

BENEFITS OF BROCCOLI:

Broccoli is a powerful, cancer-fighting cruciferous vegetable. It contains calcium and vitamin K, which both contribute to lowering the risk of bone fractures. Studies conducted on broccoli have shown its protective role against cancers of the breast, colon, liver, and prostate. The 81 milligrams of vitamin C found in one cup of broccoli exceed the recommended daily allowance of 60 milligrams per day. Since high doses of Vitamin C are required to combat illness and disease, broccoli is a great ingredient to incorporate into your regular meal plans.

Total Time: 15 min.
Serves: 2-4

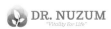

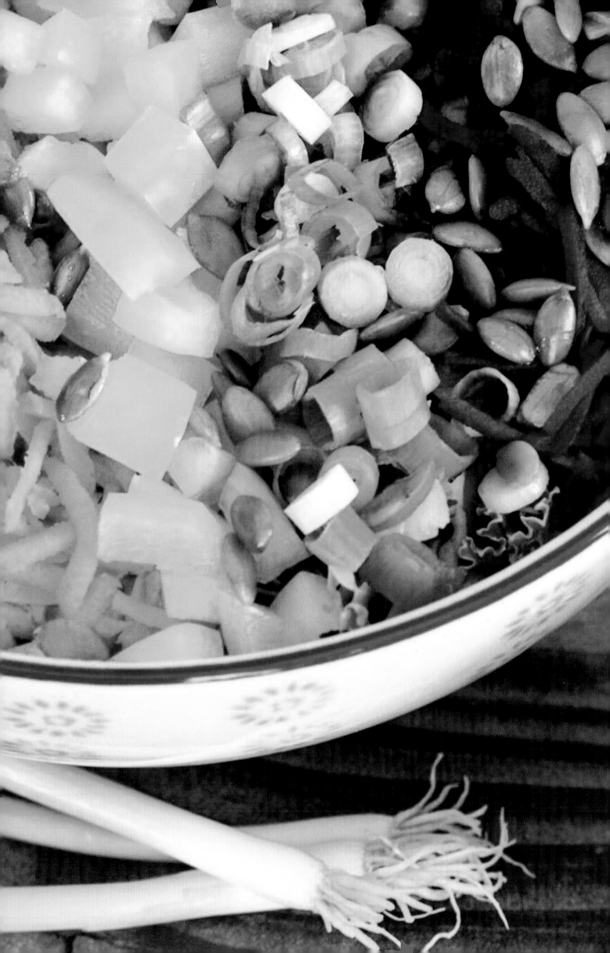

Rainbow Detox Salad

INGREDIENTS:

1/4 to 1/2 purple cabbage, chopped

4 kale leaves, chopped and stems removed

6 romaine lettuce leaves, chopped

1/2 yellow bell pepper, diced

Bundle of parsley, finely chopped

1 cup cherry tomatoes, cut in halves

2-3 green onions, sliced

1 large carrot, shredded

1 raw beet, peeled and shredded

1/2 cup pepitas

DIRECTIONS:

Add all ingredients to a large bowl. Add grilled chicken if desired.

Top with pepitas.

• • • • •

This salad can be made in so many different ways; you really can't go wrong with what you throw into it! Feel free to add, omit, or replace any vegetables in this salad.

This recipe makes a big batch, which is perfect for staying prepared and being able to take your lunch on the go.

The strawberry poppyseed vinaigrette on page 207 tastes wonderful on this salad.

BENEFITS OF GREEN ONION:

Green onions, also known as spring onions, inhibit cancer cell growth and assist in protecting the body's DNA. The sulfur compounds are anti-microbial, anti-bacterial and anti-viral, and enhance the liver's detoxification pathways. Green onions are great for immunity, support eye health, and help in lowering blood sugar levels. In Chinese Medicine, they are used to treat the common cold, ease congestion, prevent diarrhea, and improve circulation.

Total Time: 35 min.
Serves: 4-6

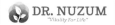

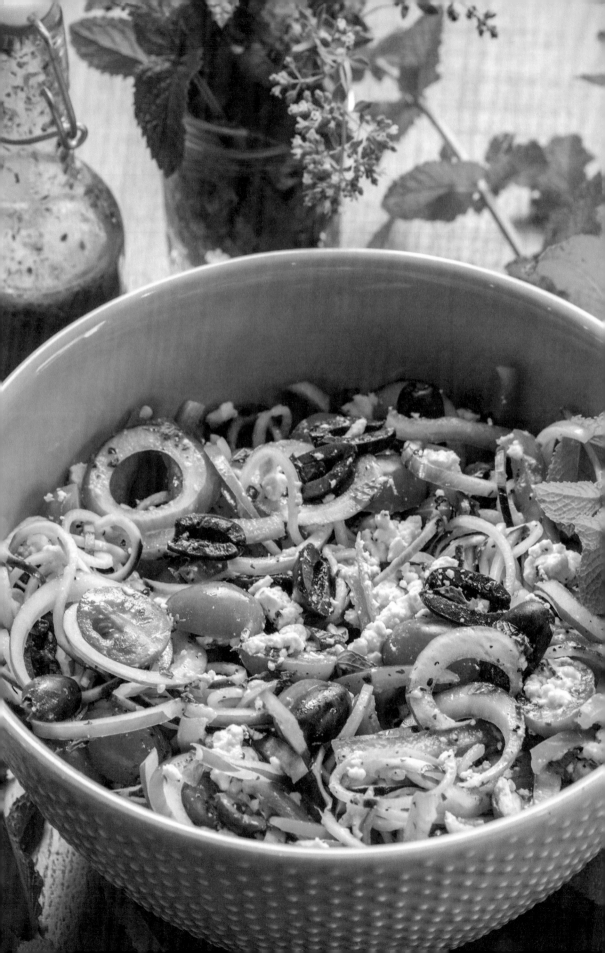

Spiralized Greek Salad

INGREDIENTS:

2 medium zucchinis

2 medium cucumbers

1/2 red onion, thinly sliced

1 bell pepper, julienned

1 cup grape tomatoes, halved

1/4 cup pitted kalamata olives, halved

4 ounces feta cheese, crumbled

DIRECTIONS:

Spiralize the zucchini and cucumber and place in a large bowl. Cut any long pieces.

Add red onion and bell peppers.

Top with tomatoes, feta cheese, and olives.

Add Greek dressing slowly, according to preference. There will be extra dressing. (See Greek Vinaigrette on page 209).

———————• • • • • •———————

This salad is so refreshing and satisfying. It's the perfect recipe to make ahead and have ready in your refrigerator for a quick lunch or dinner.

BENEFITS OF KALAMATA OLIVES:

Kalamata olives are an excellent source of vitamin A, which is important for healthy vision, immunity, and reproduction. Olives contain the "good fat"— monounsaturated—which is associated with lowering the risk of cardiovascular disease and lowering blood pressure. Olives also contain calcium, fiber, and blood-building iron, and possess a totally unique anti-oxidant and anti-inflammatory nutrient profile separate from those found in other plant foods.

Total Time: 25 min.
Serves: 6-8

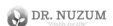

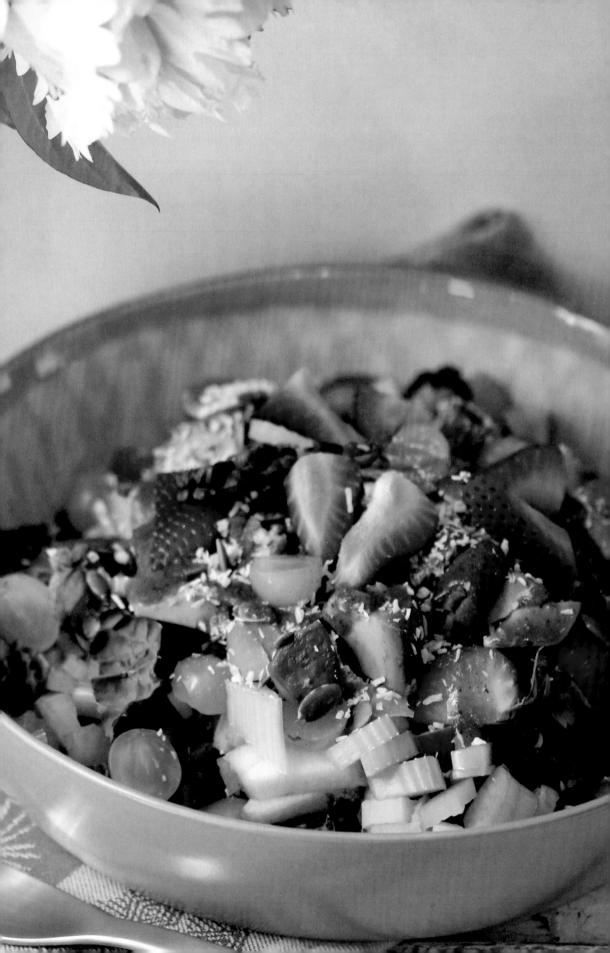

Strawberry Celery Kale Detox Salad

SALAD INGREDIENTS:

4 kale leaves, chopped in thin strips

8 large strawberries, cut into pieces (save 2 strawberries and all the strawberry leaves for dressing)

1 peeled avocado, chopped

1/2 cup grapes, halved

1 small apple or pear, chopped

4 celery stalks, chopped

1/4 cup pepitas (pumpkin seeds)

1/4 cup pecans

1 tablespoon dried, shredded coconut (for the topping)

DRESSING INGREDIENTS:

Strawberry and Leaves Dressing

Blend the following in blender:

2 whole strawberries, with leaves

1 teaspoon honey

Pinch Celtic salt

Dash ground pepper

1/4 teaspoon poppy seeds

1/4 cup olive oil

1/2 cup water

DIRECTIONS:

Toss all ingredients except coconut flakes. Mix with Strawberry and Leaves Dressing and let sit for 20 minutes to help soften the kale.

Top with coconut flakes and serve.

● ● ● ● ● ●

This salad has incredible texture and flavor. Packed with super foods, sweetness and crunch, it is sure to wake up the tastebuds and satisfy during a detox.

BENEFITS OF CELERY:

Just one stalk of celery aids in digestion, calms the nervous system, lowers blood pressure, and supplies Vitamin A for eye health. Multiple studies have confirmed that powerful flavonoids, specifically luteolin in celery, inhibit the growth of cancer cells, especially in the pancreas. Another substance in celery, apigenin, has been effective in treating breast cancer. Additional health benefits include reducing inflammation, increasing circulation, and providing relief from aches and pains.

Total Time: 10 min.
Serves: 2-4

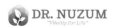

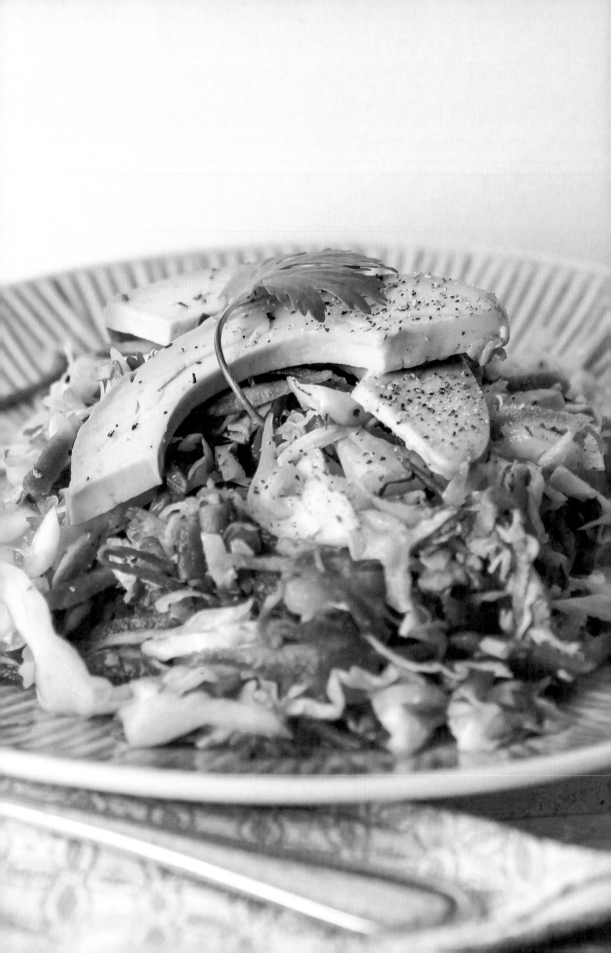

Zesty Cilantro-Lime Cabbage Salad

INGREDIENTS:

1/4 small green cabbage, thinly sliced

1/2 lime, juiced

1 bunch cilantro, chopped in small pieces (about 1/2 cup)

1 large purple carrot, shredded (or any color carrot)

1 tablespoon honey

1/2 teaspoon Celtic salt

Add pepper to taste

1 tablespoon olive oil

Avocado slices

DIRECTIONS:

Combine all ingredients and let sit for about 10 minutes.

Top with avocado slices and serve.

• • • • •

This salad is incredibly fresh and zesty—a unique cabbage salad with a Mexican cilantro-lime twist.

Sometimes cabbage can cause gas or bloating. To avoid this reaction, soak cabbage in filtered water with one tablespoon raw apple cider vinegar for 20 minutes. Then, rinse and prepare.

BENEFITS OF CABBAGE:

Most people may not think of cabbage as a nutritional powerhouse, but it is full of surprise benefits. Cabbage is actually higher in vitamin C than most citrus fruits, packed with antioxidants, and is a great food for reducing free radicals. Cabbage also has anti-inflammatory properties because of its glutamine content and is a great source of fiber to help keep the digestive system working optimally.

Total Time: 10 min.
Serves: 2-4

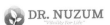

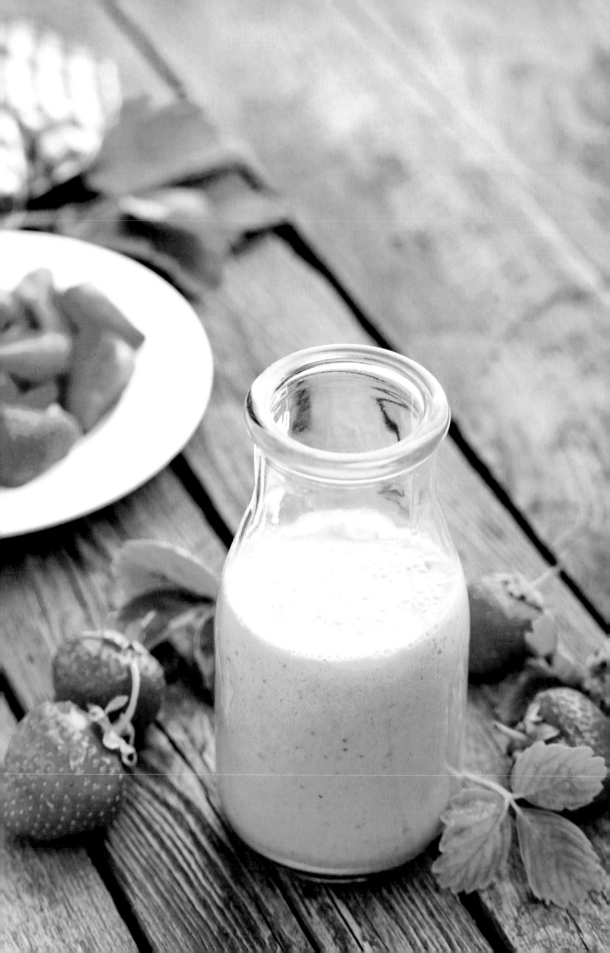

Strawberry Poppyseed Vinaigrette

INGREDIENTS:

1 cup fresh or frozen strawberries, with leaves (check for mold)

1/4 cup cold-pressed olive oil

2 tablespoons honey (unfiltered and raw)

2 tablespoons apple cider vinegar

1/4 teaspoon Himalayan pink salt

1/8 teaspoon black pepper

1/4 teaspoon poppy seeds

DIRECTIONS:

Add all ingredients, except for poppy seeds, in a high-speed blender and blend until smooth. Stir in poppy seeds and serve.

———————●••••●———————

This sweet vinaigrette is great to top any salad.

BENEFITS OF STRAWBERRY LEAVES:

Did you know that strawberry leaves are a highly nutritious part of the fruit? The leaves of strawberries are antifungal, antibacterial, and rich in vitamin C. The nutrients contained in the leaves can enhance digestion, increase mental clarity, reduce inflammation, and reduce stored fat. Here are some ways you can get these nutrient rich leaves into your diet: add them to smoothies, toss them fresh into a salad, or blend them into homemade salad dressings.

Total Time: 10 min.
Makes 2 cups

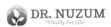

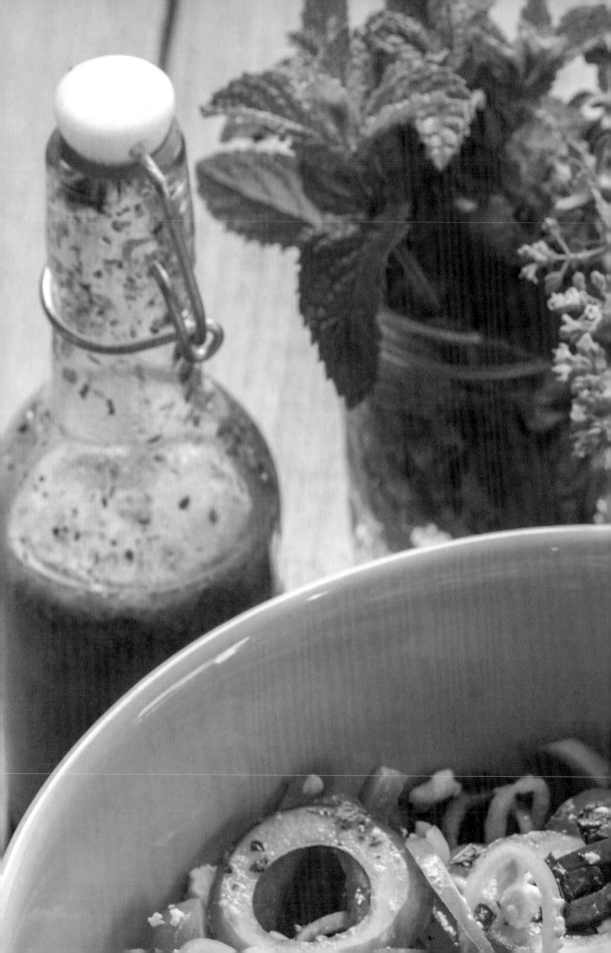

Greek Vinaigrette

INGREDIENTS:

1/2 cup olive oil

1/2 cup red wine vinegar or apple cider vinegar

1/2 lemon, juiced

1 teaspoon dijon mustard

2 teaspoons pure maple syrup or raw honey

1 garlic clove, minced

1 1/2 teaspoon dried oregano

1 1/2 teaspoon dried basil

1 teaspoon dried parsley

1 1/2 tablespoons fresh mint, finely chopped

1 teaspoon onion powder

1 teaspoon salt

1 teaspoon pepper

OPTION:

May replace dried herbs with fresh, by increasing amount to 1 1/2 tablespoon each.

DIRECTIONS:

Whisk all ingredients together until blended well. Let dressing sit for a minimum of 10 minutes to allow flavors to blend.

— • • • • • —

This dressing is perfect for the spiralized Greek Salad on page 201.

BENEFITS OF APPLE CIDER VINEGAR:

Unfiltered apple cider vinegar contains strands of proteins, enzymes, and good bacteria, referred to as "mother." The mother may be responsible for the majority of its health benefits and should be present in quality apple cider vinegar brands. Diabetics can benefit from apple cider vinegar as it improves insulin sensitivity when eating carbs, can significantly lower blood glucose responses, and may help fasting blood sugars by taking 2 tablespoons prior to going to bed. If you want to lose weight, taking a tablespoon of apple cider vinegar prior to eating may help you feel full quicker, thus reducing your overall caloric intake. Apple Cider Vinegar has a low pH which assists the stomach in breaking down protein, helping improve digestion and elimination.

> Total Time: 10 min.
> Makes 2 cups

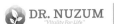

Entrées

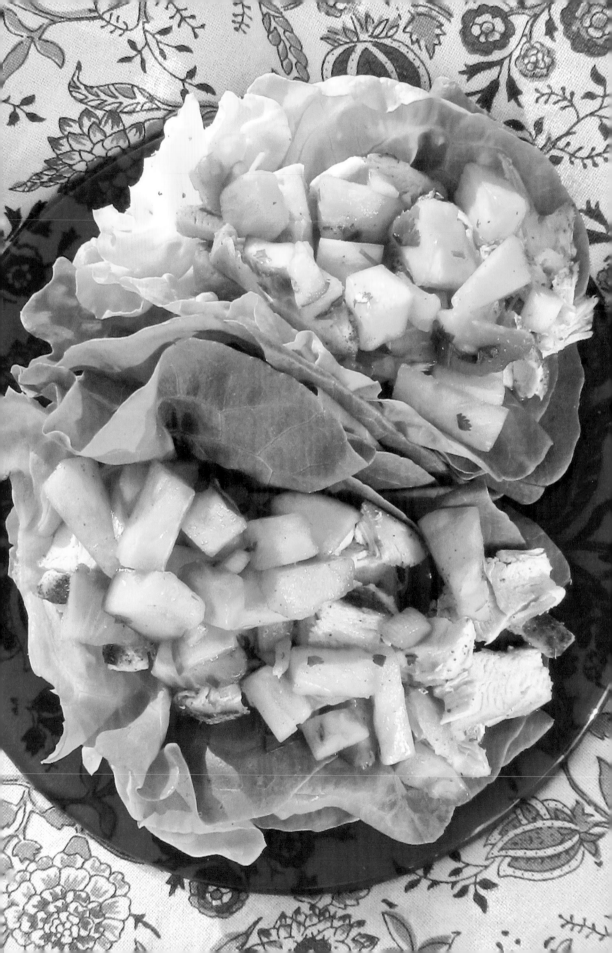

Grilled Chicken Tacos

INGREDIENTS:

1 head butter lettuce

3 organic, free-range, boneless and skinless chicken breasts

1 teaspoon cumin

1 teaspoon chili powder

3 cloves finely minced garlic

1 teaspoon Celtic salt

1/2 teaspoon ground pepper

1 tablespoon organic olive oil

1/2 lemon, juiced

DIRECTIONS:

In a glass container, combine oil, lemon juice, and spices. Mix well and then add chicken breast. Cover and place in the refrigerator for 2 hours to marinate.

Heat grill (or cast iron griddle) to medium heat. Grill on both sides until internal temperature of chicken is at least 165°.

Let rest for 5 minutes then chop or shred chicken meat.

For taco "shells," cut off the bottom of butter lettuce, gently rinse leaves, and pat dry with kitchen towel.

Use two leaves of lettuce for each taco to ensure it doesn't fall apart.

Layer chicken into lettuce shells to serve.

Top with Strawberry Pineapple Salsa from page 171.

———————• • • • • • •———————

These tasty tacos are served on butter lettuce topped with zesty strawberry pineapple salsa. This spicy, mouthwatering recipe is not only healthy but visually stunning as well. The flavors and textures of this dish will keep your palate happy during a detox. You won't even miss the corn taco shells or flour tortillas.

BENEFITS OF CHICKEN:

One of the highest sources of protein in the average person's diet, chicken is loaded with health benefits. Protein is made of amino acids, which helps build muscle. Chicken is also a great source of vitamins B and D. Vitamin B helps boost immunity, regulate digestion, and improves the nervous system. It even helps reduce gray hair! Vitamin D strengthens bones, and the iron found in chicken helps form hemoglobin, supports muscles, and fights anemia.

| Total Time: 40 min. |
| Serves: 4-6 |

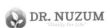

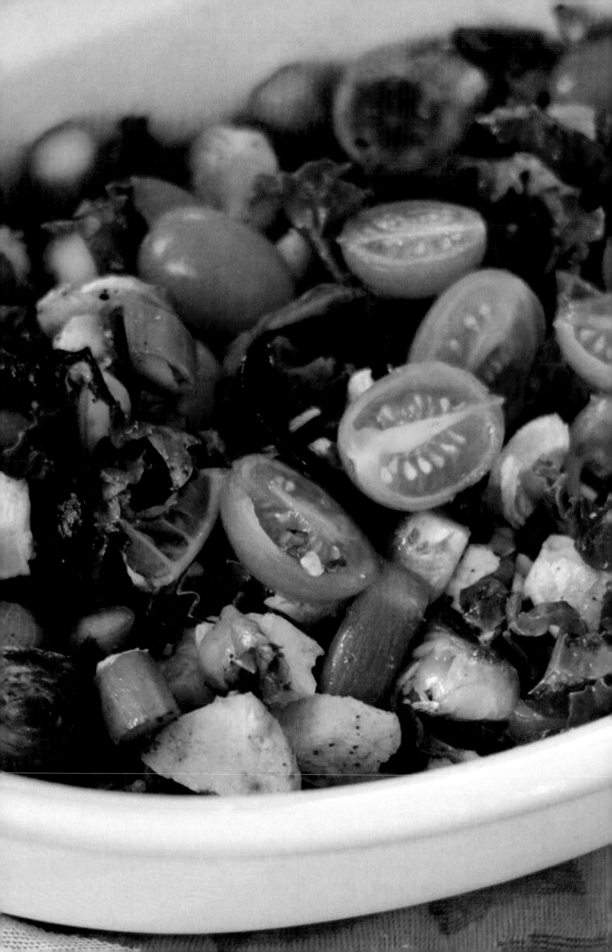

Cast Iron Chicken

INGREDIENTS:

1 chicken breast

1 tablespoon avocado oil

4 slices red onion

2 cloves garlic

1/4 teaspoon Celtic salt

8-10 asparagus spears

8 cherry tomatoes, cut in halves

1/2 bell pepper, sliced

6-10 Brussels sprouts, cut in halves

4 kale leaves, finely chopped

1 tablespoon organic cold press olive oil or avocado oil

1 tablespoon lemon juice

DIRECTIONS:

Add avocado oil to a preheated cast iron skillet on medium heat.

Season chicken breast with salt and pepper and place in skillet with two fresh garlic cloves. Cook chicken on each side until browned on both sides, approximately 5-7 minutes, or until juices of chicken run clear. Add slices of onion halfway through the cooking process to avoid burning them. Remove chicken and let it rest for 5 minutes, then cut into cubes.

Add cut vegetables, using the same cast iron skillet. Stir constantly for about 5-10 minutes on medium heat, or until peppers and asparagus start to soften. Fold chicken cubes back to your skillet with vegetables and mix together.

When serving, drizzle mixture with olive oil, lemon juice, and salt and pepper to taste.

—————→ • • • • • •————

This is a very satisfying and filling meal. For those who feel the taste of asparagus is a bit strong, it blends very well into this dish, lending a more subtle flavor that is not overpowering.

BENEFITS OF ASPARAGUS:

Asparagus is a powerful anti-inflammatory that is also high in antioxidants. It is a good source of copper, choline, fiber, folate, iron, manganese, pantothenic acid, phosphorus, potassium, thiamin, and Vitamins A, B1, B2, B3, B6, C, E and K. A five ounce serving contains 60 percent of the recommended daily allowance for folate.

| Total Time: 30 min. |
| Serves: 2 |

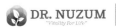

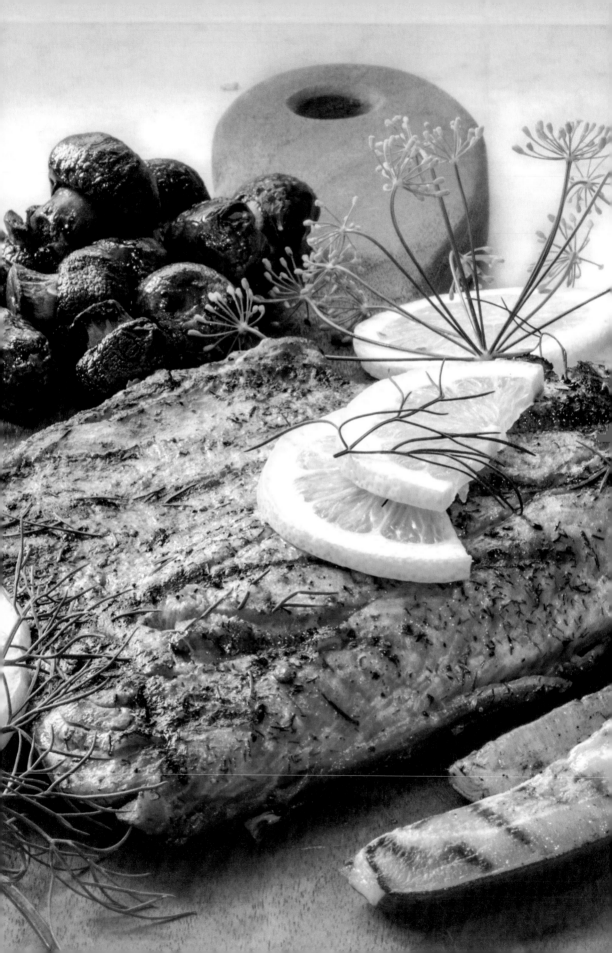

Lemon Dill Grilled Salmon

INGREDIENTS:

Side of wild-caught salmon with skin cut into 6 ounce pieces (about 5 pieces)

1/4 cup avocado oil, plus more for grill

Juice of 1 lemon

1-2 garlic cloves, minced

1 teaspoon Himalayan pink salt

1/2 teaspoon pepper

fresh dill, chopped

5 teaspoons grass-fed butter

DIRECTIONS:

Preheat grill for medium heat and brush avocado oil on grill.

In a small bowl, combine avocado oil, lemon juice, and minced garlic. Brush onto flesh and skin side.

Sprinkle salt and pepper onto salmon and then top with dill.

Place the salmon flesh side down onto grill. Allow to cook for 4 to 5 minutes per side or until salmon reaches 145-150°. Keep a close eye on the temperature—cook time may vary depending on thickness of fillets. Don't overcook the fish.

Very carefully remove fillets and add a teaspoon of butter to each fillet while still hot.

Serve immediately.

• • • • •

This dish is easy to put together and doesn't require much cooking time. Pair it with your favorite vegetables for the perfect detox meal. Be sure the salmon is wild-caught—not farmed.

BENEFITS OF WILD-CAUGHT SALMON:

Salmon is full of nutritional benefits such as vitamin B12, vitamin D, selenium, and omega-3 fatty acids—all of which are anti-inflammatory.

Total Time: 25 min.
Serves: 5

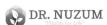

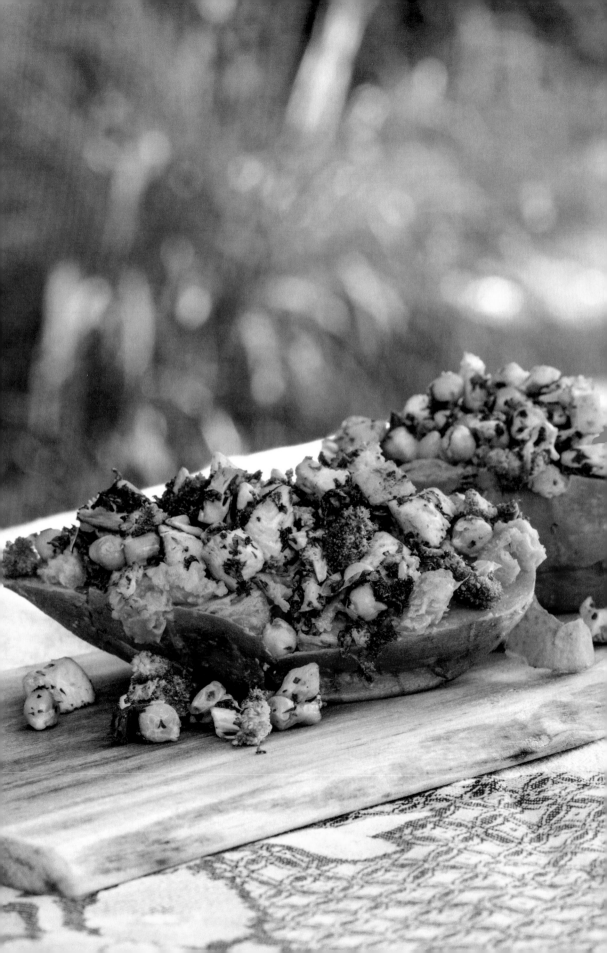

Stuffed Sweet Potatoes

INGREDIENTS:

4 small sweet potatoes or yams

2 cups kale, finely chopped

2 cups broccoli florets

3 garlic cloves, minced

2 teaspoons avocado oil

1/2 cup cooked organic chickpeas

1 large free-range chicken breast, grilled and chopped

1 lemon, juiced and zested

1 tablespoon parsley, finely chopped

1 tablespoon basil, finely chopped

1 teaspoon Himalayan pink salt

1/2 teaspoon freshly ground pepper

4 teaspoons coconut oil, divided

DIRECTIONS:

Preheat oven to 400°.

Wash sweet potatoes and pierce 2-3 times with a fork. Place on an edged baking sheet lined with parchment paper and bake for 45 minutes to an hour, or until center is cooked.

In a large sauté pan, heat avocado oil until shimmering. Add kale, broccoli, garlic, and salt and pepper. Sauté on medium-high for 5 minutes.

Add drained chickpeas, lemon juice and zest, chopped chicken, and fresh herbs. Cook for another 5 minutes then remove mixture from heat.

Slice the potato down the middle, then carefully squeeze to push it open. If your potatoes are a bit too big for one person, cut them in half length-wise.

Top with 1 teaspoon of coconut oil and a healthy scoop of the stuffing mixture.

—————● • • • • ●—————

Adding this healthy stuffing to an already nutrient dense vegetable makes this dish a perfect meal for detoxing or any time.

BENEFITS OF SWEET POTATOES:

Sweet potatoes are a great source of vitamin A, vitamin B5, B6, vitamin C, and D. They are also full of minerals such as iron, magnesium, and potassium. Additionally, sweet potatoes contain a chemical called diosgenin, a plant pyhto-estrogen, which helps to regulate hormones in both men and women.

Total Time: 90 min.
Serves: 4

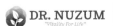

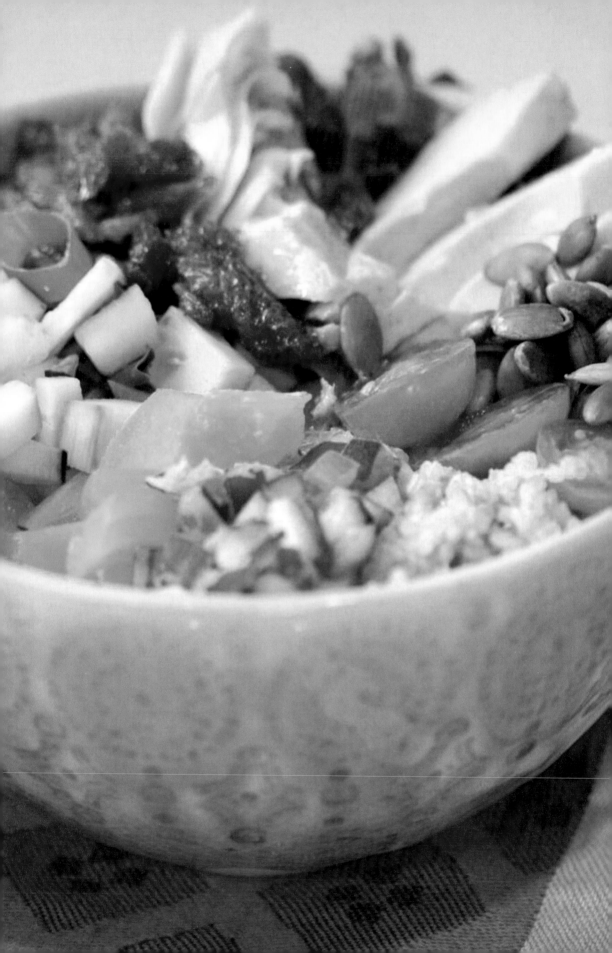

Quinoa Vegetable Bowl

INGREDIENTS:

1 1/2 cups quinoa, cooked

1 cup cherry tomatoes, cut in half

1 green onion, chopped

1/4 cup red onion, finely chopped

1/2 jar of artichokes (in water), cut in slices

1 cup kale, finely chopped

1/2 cup cilantro, finely chopped

1 bell pepper, diced

1 English cucumber, diced

1 avocado, sliced

1 lemon, juiced

3 tablespoon olive oil

DIRECTIONS:

Place ingredients into a bowl and top with avocado.

Add lemon, olive oil, and salt and pepper to taste.

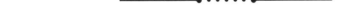

This is a very filling and delicious meal, perfect for lunch or dinner.

BENEFITS OF ARTICHOKES:

Artichokes contain an antioxidant called cynarine that reduces fat build up in the liver as well as protects the liver tissue and acts as a diuretic in the kidneys, enhancing detoxification all around.

Total Time: 25 min.
Serves: 2-3

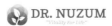

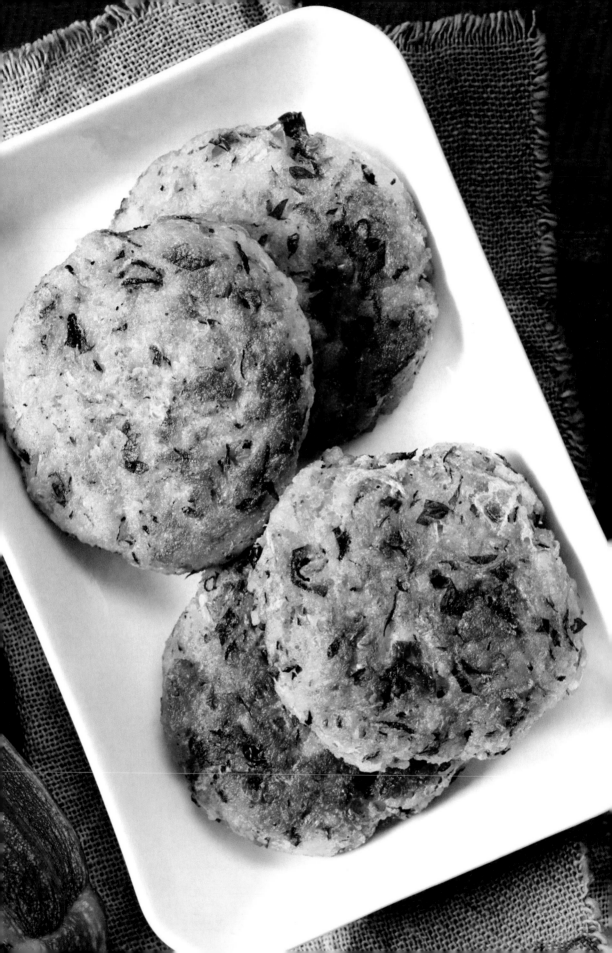

Zucchini Fritters

INGREDIENTS:

4 cups zucchini, grated

1/2 red onion, shredded

1/2 yellow pepper, finely minced

1/2 jalapeño, shredded

2 cloves garlic, finely minced

2 tablespoons basil, chopped

1 organic egg, beaten

1/3 cup coconut flour

1 teaspoon Himalayan pink salt

1/2 teaspoon ground pepper

1 teaspoon cumin

2 tablespoons avocado oil

DIRECTIONS:

Shred zucchini in food processor or with grater. Place shredded zucchini in the middle of a large piece of cheesecloth. Wrap tightly and squeeze liquid out. Let rest and press again. Repeat three to four times to ensure zucchini is dry.

Place zucchini, beaten egg, flour, red onion, peppers, garlic, basil, and salt and pepper into a mixing bowl. Mix gently but well.

Preheat the avocado oil in a large pan on medium heat. Scoop approximately one tablespoon of the mixture for each fritter and place in heated oil. Fry until fritters are golden brown, then flip and brown the other side, approximately 3-5 minutes per side. If you did not get enough water out of the zucchini the fritters may not be crisp. If so, simply bake in oven for 10 minutes at 350 degrees.

It may take a few rounds to use all the mixture, depending on the size of your pan, but you will want to use all the batter because it gets too runny after it sits.

Place on a platter lined with parchment paper. As the fritters cool they will keep their shape nicely. Serve at room temperature.

———————— • • • • • • ————————

These fritters are a great replacement for fried potatoes. They go well with eggs for breakfast and as a side to many entrées. Be sure to use avocado oil because it does not turn into a hydrogenated oil when heated to high temperatures.

BENEFITS OF BASIL:

High in cancer-fighting, disease-fighting antioxidants, basil possesses anti-inflammatory, anti-bacterial, and anti-microbial properties. Just two tablespoons of fresh chopped basil contains 27 percent of the Recommended Daily Allowance of vitamin K, which aids in healthy blood clotting. Unique, water-soluble flavonoids in basil protect cell structures and chromosomes from oxidative damage and radiation.

> Total Time: 35 min.
> Makes 6-8 fritters

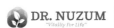

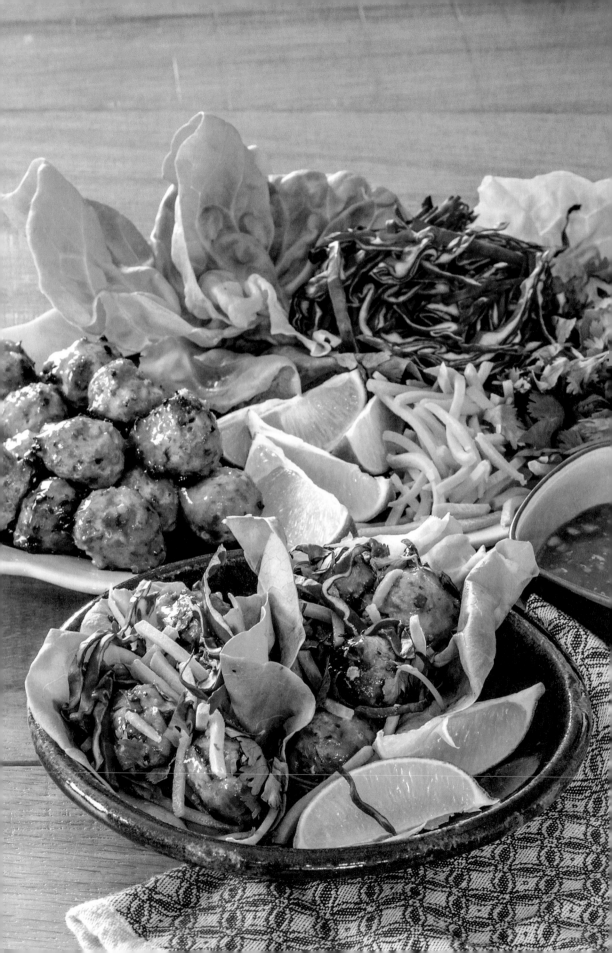

Asian Meatball Lettuce Wraps

INGREDIENTS:

Meatballs

1 1/2 pounds ground chicken

3 cloves garlic, minced

2 tablespoons ginger, minced

1/4 cup coconut aminos

1/2 cup cilantro, finely chopped

1 teaspoon chili flakes

Taco Shells and Topping

2 containers organic butter lettuce

3 carrots, shredded

1 cup purple cabbage, shredded

1 cup cilantro, chopped

2 limes cut into wedges

DIRECTIONS:

Mix meatball ingredients gently until evenly distributed. Try not to over-mix, or meatballs may be tough. Put chicken mixture in refrigerator for one hour to allow flavors to blend and to make the meatballs easier to form.

Line two baking sheets with parchment paper. Use a teaspoon or small ice cream scoop to consistently portion the mixture. Form into balls and place on prepared baking sheet. Smaller meatballs work best for lettuce wraps.

Place meatballs in a 400°, preheated oven and bake for 20 minutes, or until internal temperature is at least 165°. Carefully remove meatballs from the baking sheet and coat with Asian Sauce from page 175. Immediately place on a serving platter with extra sauce for dressing.

Remove roots, then clean butter lettuce leaves with damp paper towel. Separate lettuce leaves. Use one large leaf for base and two smaller leaves to make a sturdy wrap. Place three meatballs per wrap and top with carrots, cabbage, cilantro, and a bit of Asian sauce. Top with a squeeze of lime juice and serve.

———————•••••—•———————

These lettuce wraps have incredible flavor and satisfy the palate without compromising your health or detox. This recipe is easy to double or triple and freezes really well as long as you keep the meatballs separate from the sauce.

BENEFITS OF LETTUCE:

Low in calories and high in water volume and fiber, lettuce is an ideal detox food. Dietary fiber helps lower high cholesterol, and the potassium contained in lettuce helps lower high blood pressure. The milky white fluid that you can see when you chop or break lettuce gives it its slightly bitter taste. In Chinese medicine, bitter flavors are associated with having medicinal qualities.

| Total Time: 2 hours |
| Serves: 6 |

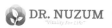

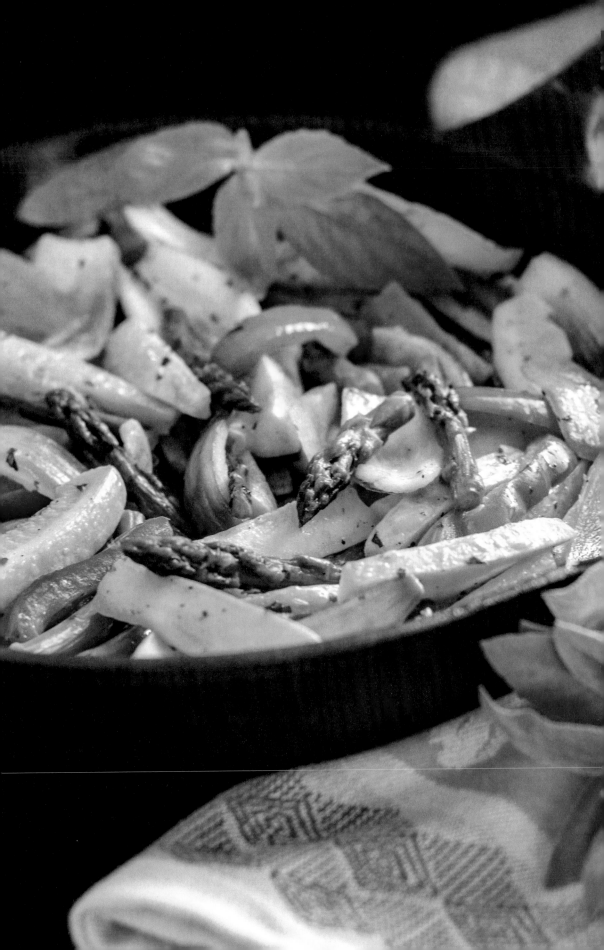

Vegetable Stir-Fry

INGREDIENTS:

1 bunch asparagus, chopped

2 yellow squash, cut in spears

1 purple onion, chopped

3 cloves garlic, finely chopped

2 tablespoons fresh herbs of your choice, chopped

1 red or orange pepper, cut in strips

2 tablespoons avocado oil

Salt and pepper to taste

Half a lemon, juiced

DIRECTIONS:

Prepare all vegetables and herbs and mix together in large bowl.

Heat oil on high heat in a large skillet or stir-fry pan. Add vegetable mixture to pan, stirring quickly for five minutes, or until vegetables become slightly tender. Keep the color bright and texture firm.

Garnish with fresh herbs and a squeeze of lemon.

● ● ● ● ● ●

This simple dish is colorful, flavorful, and satisfying as either a side or an entrée. It can be put together quickly and can even be made ahead of time.

BENEFITS OF PURPLE ONION:

Purple onions contain important flavonoids that help lower cancer risk as well as neutralize free radicals, protecting vital organs. Onions also contain biotin, manganese, copper, vitamin B6, vitamin C, fiber, phosphorus, potassium, vitamin B1, and folate. Peel as little of the outer layer off as possible, since the flavonoids tend to be concentrated in and near the outer portion.

| Total Time: 10 min. |
| Serves: 4 |

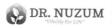

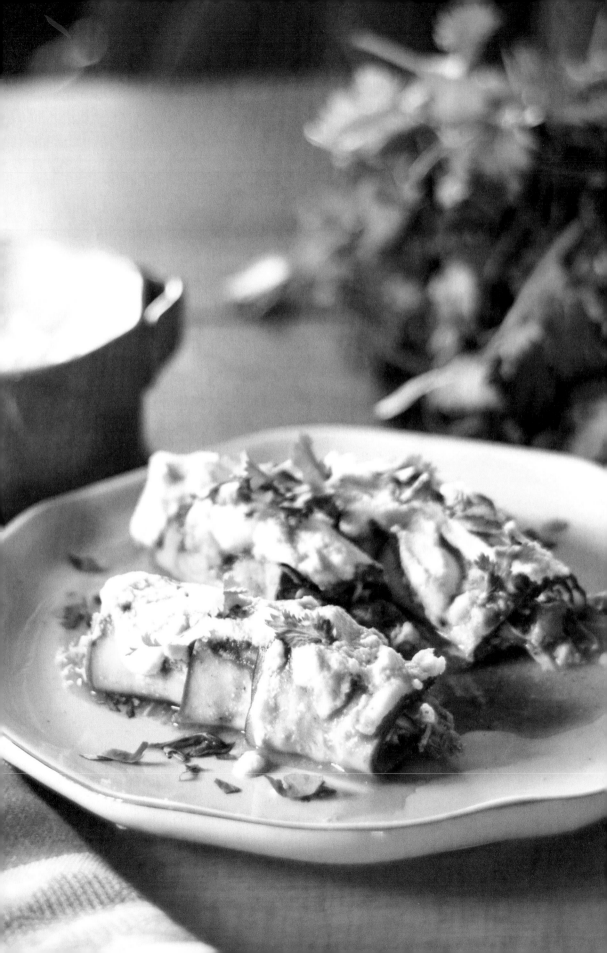

Zucchini Enchiladas

INGREDIENTS:

4 zucchinis, washed

2 cups chicken, cooked and shredded

1/2 white onion, finely chopped

Handful of cilantro, finely chopped

1 teaspoon salt

1/2 teaspoon pepper

1 cup red chile sauce

1 cup cashew crema

DIRECTIONS:

Lay zucchini flat on cutting board and cut off both ends. Carefully pull vegetable peeler down the length of the zucchini to yield long strips. These are your tortillas for the recipe, so be careful to make whole pieces. Set strips aside.

Place shredded chicken in a medium bowl with onion, cilantro, salt, pepper, and a half-cup of red chili sauce. Stir until combined.

Slightly overlap three strips of zucchini to create the tortilla for the enchilada. Spread a spoonful of chicken across the middle of the overlapped zucchini and fold as if making regular enchiladas. Take your time and roll tight, tucking the chicken in neatly. Place rolled enchilada in baking pan and repeat with remaining zucchini slices.

Spoon red chili sauce over each enchilada, then top with cashew crema. Both recipes are found on the next page.

Cover with a lid or parchment and bake at 350°F for 25 minutes.

● ● ● ● ● ●

This recipe comes together quickly and can be made ahead and baked right before dinner. This dish will take your mind right to your favorite Mexican restaurant, and you will feel none of the guilt or side effects of eating toxic food.

BENEFITS OF ZUCCHINI:

Zucchini may be one of the most nutrient rich varieties of summer squash. It contains vitamin A, magnesium, folate, potassium, copper, and phosphorus. Zucchini is also a great source of omega-3 fatty acids, zinc, niacin, and protein. Finally, this squash is great for maintaining overall health as it is rich in vitamin B1, vitamin B6, vitamin B2, and calcium. In Chinese medicine, zucchini is used to rid the body of intestinal parasites.

Total Time: 1 hour
Serves: 4

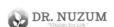

Red Chile Sauce

INGREDIENTS:

6 dried Mexican chilies (preferably large anaheim or hatch chilies if available)

2 cups water

2 tablespoons coconut oil

3 fresh tomatoes, chopped

3 garlic cloves

Handful of cilantro, chopped

1 teaspoon of salt

1/2 teaspoon pepper

DIRECTIONS:

Prep chilies by taking off stems and shaking out seeds. Toast chilies on each side in a medium sized frying pan, until chilies become fragrant.

Pour two cups water over the chilies and simmer on medium heat for 15 minutes. Weigh down the chilies with a glass plate to submerge them in the water.

Add tomatoes, garlic, cilantro, garlic, salt, and pepper to high-speed blender. Carefully add chilies and the juice. Put blender lid on tight and slowly turn up the speed. Be extremely careful while using hot liquid in a blender. Blend until chilies are completely broken down. If you do not have a powerful blender, let the chilies cool and pour mixture through a sieve to separate the chili puree from the skins.

Return sauce to pan and add coconut oil. Let the mixture simmer for 30 minutes on medium heat and stir every few minutes. It takes quite a bit of salt to flavor red chili, so more than one teaspoon may be required. Add more water if you feel the sauce is too thick.

The sauce will store in the refrigerator for seven days and freezes well.

———————• • • • • •———————

This chile sauce goes well with any Mexican dish, but is particularly delicious on the zucchini enchiladas on the previous page.

BENEFITS OF RED CHILES:

Red chiles contain Vitamins C, A, and cancer fighting lycopene. Chiles can help reduce pain and are powerful anti-oxidants that can ease symptoms of colds and flu. Ancient remedies have put red chiles and chile powder to use as a preventative for heart attacks.

Total Time: 30 min.
Makes 3-4 cups

Cashew Crema

INGREDIENTS:

1 cup cashews, soaked

5-7 tablespoons water

2-4 drops apple cider vinegar

1 lime, juiced

Salt to taste

DIRECTIONS:

Soak cashews in filtered water for 2 hours, then drain.

Add all ingredients to high-speed blender and blend on high for 2 minutes.

If mixture is too thick, add one tablespoon of water at a time until desired consistency is achieved.

Top enchiladas prior to baking with half of the mixture. Serve remaining crema as a condiment.

● • • • • ●

The cream sauce will add a richness to a dish that cheese would normally add, but the cashew sauce is so much better for you!

BENEFITS OF CASHEWS:

Cashews contain magnesium which aids over 300 biological processes in the body, including keeping your heart healthy. Cashews also contain vitamins, anti-oxidants, and the good fat that keeps weight in check and satisfies the appetite. Clinical studies have shown the benefits of cashews as a remedy for depression because of healthy fats and positive effects on the brain.

Total Time: 2 hours 10 min.
Makes 2 cups

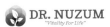